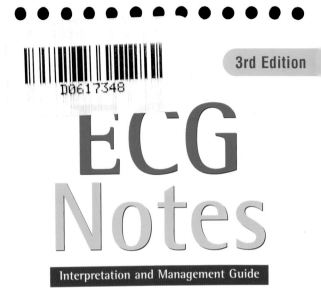

3rd Edition

ECG
Notes

Interpretation and Management Guide

Shirley A. Jones, MS Ed, MHA, MSN, EMT-P, RN

Purchase additional copies of this book at your health science bookstore or directly from F.A. Davis by shopping online at www.fadavis.com or by calling 800-323-3555 (US) or 800-665-1148 (CAN)

A Davis's Notes Book

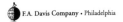

F.A. Davis Company • Philadelphia

F. A. Davis Company
1915 Arch Street
Philadelphia, PA 19103
www.fadavis.com

Printed in China by Imago

Last digit indicates print number: 10 9 8 7 6 5 4

Publisher, Nursing: Lisa B. Houck
Content Project Manager: Julia Curcio
Design and Illustration Manager: Carolyn O'Brien
Reviewers: Jill M. Mayo, RN, MSN, ACLS; Jill Scott, RN, MSN, CCRN; Patricia Sweeney, MS, CRNP, FNP, BC; Barbara Tacinelli, RN, MA

As new scientific information becomes available through basic and clinical research, recommended treatments and drug therapies undergo changes. The author(s) and publisher have done everything possible to make this book accurate, up to date, and in accord with accepted standards at the time of publication. The author(s), editors, and publisher are not responsible for errors or omissions or for consequences from application of the book, and make no warranty, expressed or implied, in regard to the contents of the book. Any practice described in this book should be applied by the reader in accordance with professional standards of care used in regard to the unique circumstances that may apply in each situation. The reader is advised always to check product information (package inserts) for changes and new information regarding dose and contraindications before administering any drug. Caution is especially urged when using new or infrequently ordered drugs.

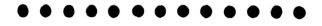

✓HIPAA compliant
✓OSHA compliant

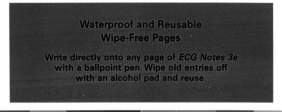

Waterproof and Reusable
Wipe-Free Pages

Write directly onto any page of *ECG Notes 3e*
with a ballpoint pen. Wipe old entries off
with an alcohol pad and reuse.

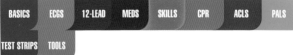

| BASICS | ECGS | 12-LEAD | MEDS | SKILLS | CPR | ACLS | PALS |

| TEST STRIPS | TOOLS |

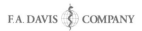

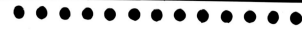

Anatomy of the Heart

The heart, a fist-sized muscular organ located in the mediastinum, is the central structure of the cardiovascular system. It is protected by the bony structures of the sternum anteriorly, the spinal column posteriorly, and the rib cage. The heart is roughly conical, with the base of the cone at the top of the heart and the apex (the pointed part) at the bottom. It is rotated slightly counterclockwise, with the apex tipped anteriorly so that the back surface of the heart actually lies over the diaphragm.

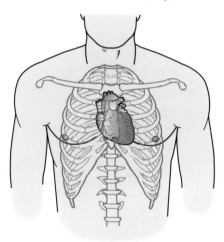

Location of the heart

♥ **Clinical Tip:** The cone-shaped heart has its tip (apex) just above the diaphragm to the left of the midline. This is why we may think of the heart as being on the left side—the strongest beat can be heard or felt there.

Layers of the Heart

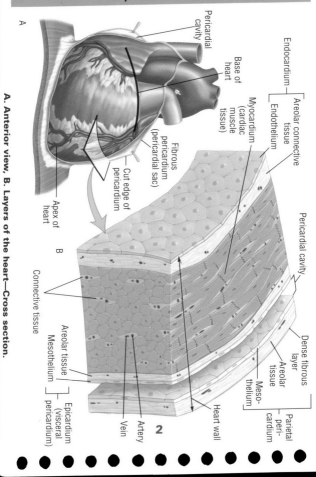

A

Pericardial cavity

Base of heart

Endocardium { Areolar connective tissue / Endothelium

Myocardium (cardiac muscle tissue)

Fibrous pericardium (pericardial sac)

Cut edge of pericardium

Apex of heart

Pericardial cavity

B

Connective tissue

Areolar tissue / Mesothelium } Epicardium (visceral pericardium)

Vein

Artery

Dense fibrous layer / Areolar tissue } Parietal pericardium

Meso-thelium

Heart wall

2

A. Anterior view, B. Layers of the heart—Cross section.

Heart—Anterior Surface

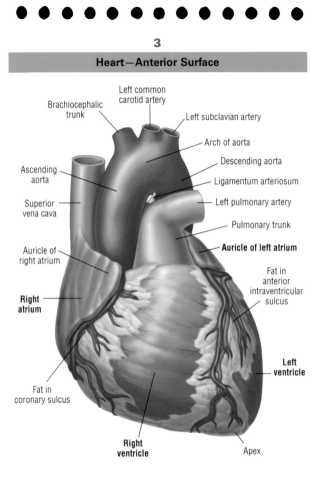

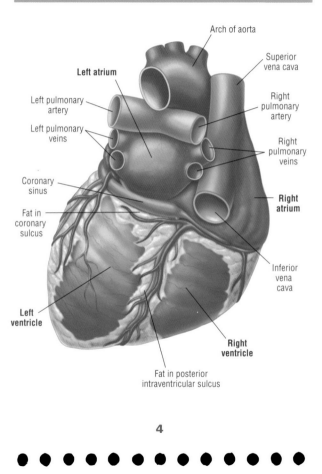

Arch of aorta

Left atrium

Left pulmonary artery

Left pulmonary veins

Coronary sinus

Fat in coronary sulcus

Left ventricle

Superior vena cava

Right pulmonary artery

Right pulmonary veins

Right atrium

Inferior vena cava

Right ventricle

Fat in posterior intraventricular sulcus

Heart—Anterior Section (arrows show direction of blood flow)

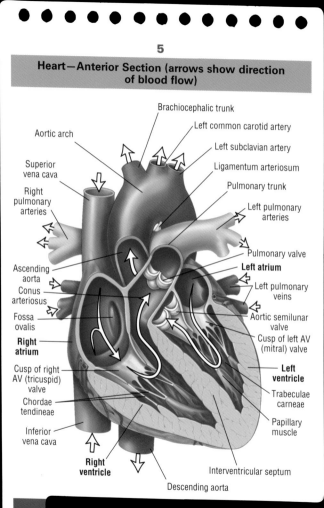

- Brachiocephalic trunk
- Left common carotid artery
- Aortic arch
- Left subclavian artery
- Superior vena cava
- Ligamentum arteriosum
- Right pulmonary arteries
- Pulmonary trunk
- Left pulmonary arteries
- Ascending aorta
- Pulmonary valve
- Conus arteriosus
- **Left atrium**
- Fossa ovalis
- Left pulmonary veins
- **Right atrium**
- Aortic semilunar valve
- Cusp of right AV (tricuspid) valve
- Cusp of left AV (mitral) valve
- Chordae tendineae
- **Left ventricle**
- Inferior vena cava
- Trabeculae carneae
- Papillary muscle
- **Right ventricle**
- Interventricular septum
- Descending aorta

Heart Valves

Properties of Heart Valves
- Fibrous connective tissue prevents enlargement of valve openings and anchors valve flaps.
- Valve closure prevents backflow of blood during and after contraction.

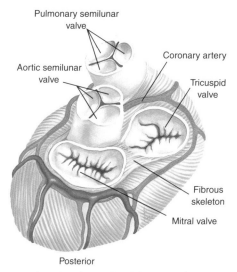

Pulmonary semilunar valve

Coronary artery

Aortic semilunar valve

Tricuspid valve

Fibrous skeleton

Mitral valve

Posterior

Superior view with atria removed

Coronary Arteries and Veins

The coronary arteries and veins provide blood to the heart muscle and the electrical conduction system. The left and right coronary arteries are the first to branch off the aorta, just above the leaflets of the aortic valve.

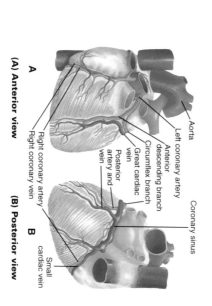

(A) Anterior view

(B) Posterior view

A

B

Aorta

Left coronary artery

Anterior descending branch

Circumflex branch

Great cardiac vein

Posterior artery and vein

Right coronary artery
Right coronary vein

Coronary sinus

Small cardiac vein

Anatomy of the Cardiovascular System

The cardiovascular system is a closed system consisting of the heart and all the blood vessels. Arteries and veins are connected by smaller structures that transport substances needed for cellular metabolism to body systems and remove the waste products of metabolism from those same tissues. Arteries carry blood away from the heart and, with the exception of the pulmonary arteries, transport oxygenated blood. Veins move blood toward the heart. With the exception of the pulmonary veins, they carry blood that is low in oxygen and high in carbon dioxide.

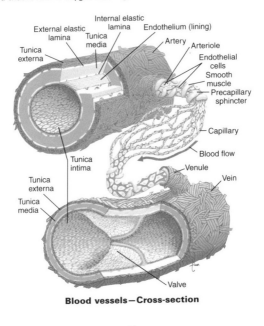

Blood vessels—Cross-section

Cardiovascular System—Major Arteries

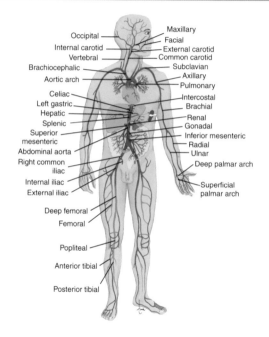

Occipital
Internal carotid
Vertebral
Brachiocephalic
Aortic arch
Celiac
Left gastric
Hepatic
Splenic
Superior mesenteric
Abdominal aorta
Right common iliac
Internal iliac
External iliac
Deep femoral
Femoral
Popliteal
Anterior tibial
Posterior tibial

Maxillary
Facial
External carotid
Common carotid
Subclavian
Axillary
Pulmonary
Intercostal
Brachial
Renal
Gonadal
Inferior mesenteric
Radial
Ulnar
Deep palmar arch
Superficial palmar arch

Cardiovascular System—Major Veins

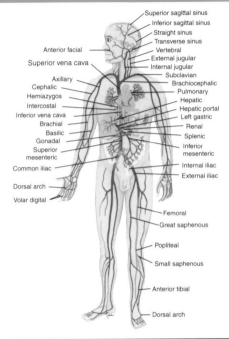

Superior sagittal sinus
Inferior sagittal sinus
Straight sinus
Transverse sinus
Vertebral
External jugular
Internal jugular
Subclavian
Brachiocephalic
Pulmonary
Hepatic
Hepatic portal
Left gastric
Renal
Splenic
Inferior mesenteric
Internal iliac
External iliac

Anterior facial
Superior vena cava
Axillary
Cephalic
Hemiazygos
Intercostal
Inferior vena cava
Brachial
Basilic
Gonadal
Superior mesenteric
Common iliac
Dorsal arch
Volar digital

Femoral
Great saphenous
Popliteal
Small saphenous
Anterior tibial
Dorsal arch

Physiology of the Heart

Normal blood flow through the heart begins at the right atrium, which receives systemic venous blood from the superior and inferior venae cavae. Blood passes from the right atrium, across the tricuspid valve, to the right ventricle. It is then pumped across the pulmonary valve into the pulmonary arteries.

Outside the heart, the left and right pulmonary arteries distribute blood to the lungs for gas exchange in the pulmonary capillaries. Oxygenated blood returns to the left atrium through the left and right pulmonary veins. After passing across the mitral valve, blood enters the left ventricle, where it is pumped across the aortic valve, through the aorta, and into the coronary arteries and the peripheral circulation.

Mechanics of Heart Function	
Process	**Action**
Cardiac cycle	Sequence of events in 1 heartbeat. Blood is pumped through the entire cardiovascular system.
Systole	Contraction phase—usually refers to ventricular contraction.
Diastole	Relaxation phase—the atria and ventricles are filling. Lasts longer than systole.
Stroke volume (SV)	Amount of blood ejected from either ventricle in a single contraction. Starling's Law of the Heart states that the degree of cardiac muscle stretch can increase the force of ejected blood. More blood filling the ventricles increases SV.
Cardiac output (CO)	Amount of blood pumped through the cardiovascular system per min. CO = SV × Heart rate (HR).

Properties of Cardiac Cells	
Property	**Ability**
Automaticity	Generates electrical impulse independently, without involving the nervous system.
Excitability	Responds to electrical stimulation.
Conductivity	Passes or propagates electrical impulses from cell to cell.
Contractility	Shortens in response to electrical stimulation.

Systolic and Diastolic Phases in the Heart

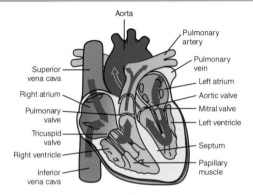

Diastole

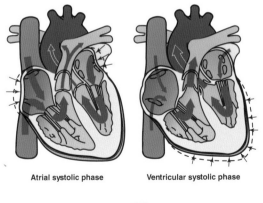

Atrial systolic phase

Ventricular systolic phase

Electrical Conduction System of the Heart

Electrophysiology	
Structure	**Function and Location**
Sinoatrial (SA or sinus) node	Dominant pacemaker of the heart, located in upper portion of right atrium. Intrinsic rate 60–100 bpm.
Internodal pathways	Direct electrical impulses between the SA and AV nodes and spread them across the atrial muscle.
Atrioventricular (AV) node	Part of the AV junctional tissue, which includes some surrounding tissue plus the connected bundle of His. The AV node slows conduction, creating a slight delay before electrical impulses are carried to the ventricles. The intrinsic rate is 40–60 bpm.
Bundle of His	At the top of the interventricular septum, this bundle of fibers extends directly from the AV node and transmits impulses to the bundle branches.
Left bundle branch	Conducts electrical impulses to the left ventricle.
Right bundle branch	Conducts electrical impulses to the right ventricle.
Purkinje system	The bundle branches terminate with this network of fibers, which spread electrical impulses rapidly throughout the ventricular walls. The intrinsic rate is 20–40 bpm.

Electrophysiology	
Action	**Effect**
Depolarization	The electrical charge of a cell is altered by a shift of electrolytes on either side of the cell membrane. This change stimulates muscle fiber to contract.
Repolarization	Chemical pumps re-establish an internal negative charge as the cells return to their resting state.

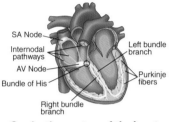

SA Node

Internodal pathways

AV Node

Bundle of His

Right bundle branch

Left bundle branch

Purkinje fibers

Conduction system of the heart

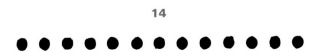

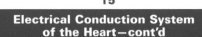

Electrical Conduction System of the Heart—cont'd

The Depolarization Process

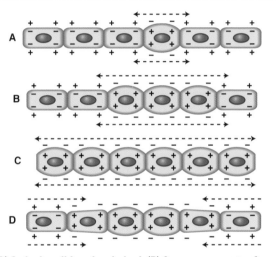

(A) A single cell has depolarized. (B) A wave propagates from cell to cell. (C) Wave propagation stops when all cells are depolarized. (D) Repolarization restores each cell's normal polarity.

Progression of Depolarization Through the Heart

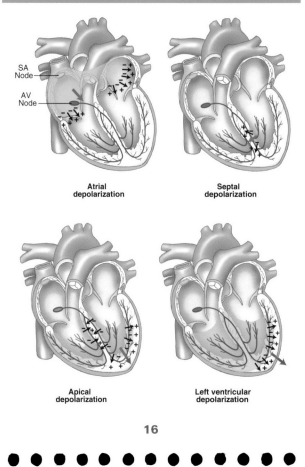

SA Node

AV Node

Atrial depolarization

Septal depolarization

Apical depolarization

Left ventricular depolarization

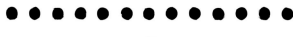

Correlation of Depolarization and Repolarization With the ECG

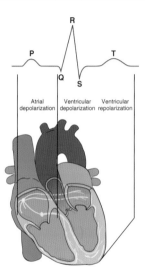

♥ **Clinical Tip:** Mechanical and electrical functions of the heart are influenced by proper electrolyte balance. Important components of this balance are sodium, calcium, potassium, and magnesium.

The Electrocardiogram (ECG)

The body acts as a giant conductor of electrical current. Electrical activity that originates in the heart can be detected on the body's surface through an electrocardiogram (ECG). Electrodes are applied to the skin to measure voltage changes in the cells between the electrodes. These voltage changes are amplified and visually displayed on an oscilloscope and graph paper.

- An ECG is a series of waves and deflections recording the heart's electrical activity from a certain "view."
- Many views, each called a lead, monitor voltage changes between electrodes placed in different positions on the body.
- Leads I, II, and III are bipolar leads and consist of two electrodes of opposite polarity (positive and negative). The third (ground) electrode minimizes electrical activity from other sources.
- Leads aVR, aVL, and aVF are unipolar leads and consist of a single positive electrode and a reference point (with zero electrical potential) that lies in the center of the heart's electrical field.
- Leads V_1–V_6 are unipolar leads and consist of a single positive electrode with a negative reference point found at the electrical center of the heart.
- An ECG tracing looks different in each lead because the recorded angle of electrical activity changes with each lead. Different angles allow a more accurate perspective than a single one would.
- The ECG machine can be adjusted to make any skin electrode positive or negative. The polarity depends on which lead the machine is recording.
- A cable attached to the patient is divided into several different-colored wires: three, four, or five for monitoring purposes, or ten for a 12-lead ECG.
- Incorrect placement of electrodes may turn a normal ECG tracing into an abnormal one.

♥ **Clinical Tip:** It is important to keep in mind that the ECG shows only electrical activity; it tells us nothing about how well the heart is working mechanically.

♥ **Clinical Tip:** Patients should be treated according to their symptoms, not merely their ECG.

♥ **Clinical Tip:** To obtain a 12-lead ECG, four wires are attached to each limb, and six wires are attached at different locations on the chest. The total of ten wires provides 12 views (12 leads).

Limb Leads

Electrodes are placed on the right arm (RA), left arm (LA), right leg (RL), and left leg (LL). With only four electrodes, six leads are viewed. These leads include the standard leads—I, II, and III—and the augmented leads—aVR, aVL, and aVF.

Standard Limb Lead Electrode Placement

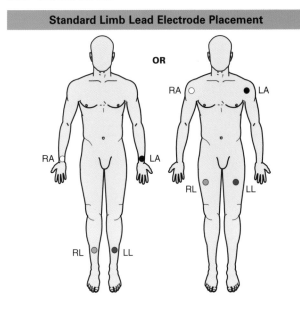

Standard Limb Leads

Leads I, II, and III make up the standard leads. If electrodes are placed on the right arm, left arm, and left leg, three leads are formed. If an imaginary line is drawn between each of these electrodes, an axis is formed between each pair of leads. The axes of these three leads form an equilateral triangle with the heart in the center (Einthoven's triangle).

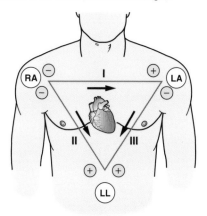

Elements of Standard Limb Leads			
Lead	Positive Electrode	Negative Electrode	View of Heart
I	LA	RA	Lateral
II	LL	RA	Inferior
III	LL	LA	Inferior

♥ **Clinical Tip:** Lead II is commonly called a monitoring lead. It provides information on heart rate, regularity, conduction time, and ectopic beats. The presence or location of an acute myocardial infarction (MI) should be further diagnosed with a 12-lead ECG.

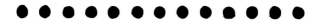
Augmented Limb Leads

Leads aVR, aVL, and aVF make up the augmented leads. Each letter of an augmented lead refers to a specific term: a = augmented; V = voltage; R = right arm; L = left arm; F = foot (the left foot).

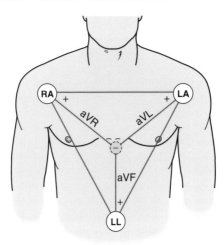

Elements of Augmented Limb Leads		
Lead	**Positive Electrode**	**View of Heart**
aVR	RA	None
aVL	LA	Lateral
aVF	LL	Inferior

Chest Leads

Standard Chest Lead Electrode Placement

The chest leads are identified as V_1, V_2, V_3, V_4, V_5, and V_6. Each electrode placed in a "V" position is positive.

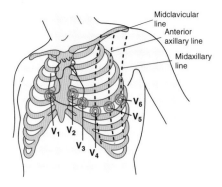

Elements of Chest Leads		
Lead	Positive Electrode Placement	View of Heart
V_1	4th Intercostal space to right of sternum	Septum
V_2	4th Intercostal space to left of sternum	Septum
V_3	Directly between V_2 and V_4	Anterior
V_4	5th Intercostal space at left midclavicular line	Anterior
V_5	Level with V_4 at left anterior axillary line	Lateral
V_6	Level with V_5 at left midaxillary line	Lateral

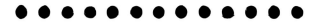

Electrode Placement Using a 3-Wire Cable

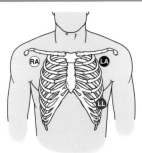

Electrode Placement Using a 5-Wire Cable

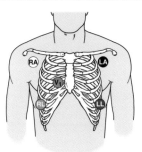

♥ **Clinical Tip:** Five-wire telemetry units are commonly used to monitor leads I, II, II, aVR, aVL, aVF, and V_1 in critical care settings.

Modified Chest Leads

- Modified chest leads (MCL) are useful in detecting bundle branch blocks and premature beats.
- Lead MCL_1 simulates chest lead V_1 and views the ventricular septum.
- Lead MCL_6 simulates chest lead V_6 and views the lateral wall of the left ventricle.

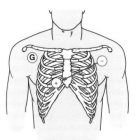

Lead MCL₁ electrode placement

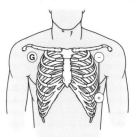

Lead MCL₆ electrode placement

♥ **Clinical Tip:** Write on the rhythm strip which simulated lead was used.

24

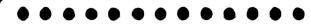
The Right-Sided 12-Lead ECG

- The limb leads are placed as usual, but the chest leads are a mirror image of the standard 12-lead chest placement.
- The ECG machine cannot recognize that the leads have been reversed. It will still print "V_1–V_6" next to the tracing. Be sure to cross this out and write the new lead positions on the ECG paper.

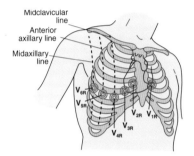

The Right-Sided 12-Lead ECG	
Chest Leads	**Position**
V_{1R}	4th Intercostal space to left of sternum
V_{2R}	4th Intercostal space to right of sternum
V_{3R}	Directly between V_{2R} and V_{4R}
V_{4R}	5th Intercostal space at right midclavicular line
V_{5R}	Level with V_{4R} at right anterior axillary line
V_{6R}	Level with V_{5R} at right midaxillary line

♥ **Clinical Tip:** Patients with an acute inferior MI should have right-sided ECGs to assess for possible right ventricular infarction.

The 15-Lead ECG

Areas of the heart that are not well visualized by the six chest leads include the wall of the right ventricle and the posterior wall of the left ventricle. A 15-lead ECG, which includes the standard 12 leads plus leads V_{4R}, V_8, and V_9, increases the chance of detecting an MI in these areas.

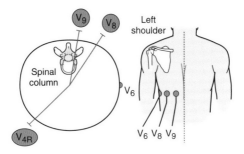

The 15-Lead ECG		
Chest Leads	**Electrode Placement**	**View of Heart**
V_{4R}	5th Intercostal space in right anterior midclavicular line	Right ventricle
V_8	Posterior 5th intercostal space in left midscapular line	Posterior wall of left ventricle
V_9	Directly between V_8 and spinal column at posterior 5th intercostal space	Posterior wall of left ventricle

♥ **Clinical Tip:** Use a 15-lead ECG when the 12-lead is normal but the history is still suggestive of an acute infarction.

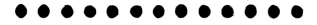

Recording of the ECG

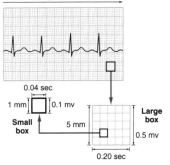

Constant speed of 25 mm/sec

0.04 sec

1 mm | 0.1 mv

Small box

Large box

5 mm

0.5 mv

0.20 sec

Components of an ECG Tracing

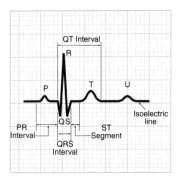

QT Interval

R

P

T

U

Isoelectric line

PR Interval

QS

ST Segment

QRS Interval

Electrical Activity	
Term	**Definition**
Wave	A deflection, either positive or negative, away from the baseline (isoelectric line) of the ECG tracing
Complex	Several waves
Segment	A straight line between waves or complexes
Interval	A segment and a wave

♥ **Clinical Tip:** Between waves and cycles, the ECG records a baseline (isoelectric line), which indicates the absence of net electrical activity.

Electrical Components	
Deflection	**Description**
P Wave	First wave seen Small, rounded, upright (positive) wave indicating atrial depolarization (and contraction)
PR Interval	Distance between beginning of P wave and beginning of QRS complex Measures time during which a depolarization wave travels from the atria to the ventricles
QRS Complex	Three deflections following P wave Indicates ventricular depolarization (and contraction) Q Wave: First negative deflection R Wave: First positive deflection S Wave: First negative deflection after R wave
ST Segment	Distance between S wave and beginning of T wave Measures time between ventricular depolarization and beginning of repolarization
T Wave	Rounded upright (positive) wave following QRS Represents ventricular repolarization
QT Interval	Distance between beginning of QRS to end of T wave Represents total ventricular activity
U Wave	Small rounded, upright wave following T wave Most easily seen with a slow HR Represents repolarization of Purkinje fibers

Methods for Calculating Heart Rate

Heart rate is the number of times the heart beats per minute (bpm). On an ECG tracing, bpm is usually calculated as the number of QRS complexes. Included are extra beats, such as premature ventricular contractions (PVCs), premature atrial contractions (PACs), and premature junctional contractions (PJCs). The rate is measured from the R-R interval, the distance between one R wave and the next. If the atrial rate (the number of P waves) and the ventricular rate (the number of QRS complexes) vary, the analysis may show them as different rates, one atrial and one ventricular. The method chosen to calculate HR varies according to rate and regularity on the ECG tracing.

Method 1: Count Large Boxes

Regular rhythms can be quickly determined by counting the number of large graph boxes between two R waves. That number is divided into 300 to calculate bpm. The rates for the first one to six large boxes can be easily memorized. Remember: 60 sec/min divided by 0.20 sec/large box = 300 large boxes/min.

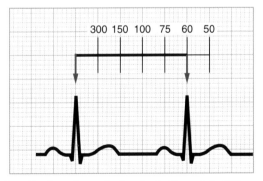

Counting large boxes for heart rate. The rate is 60 bpm.

Method 2: Count Small Boxes

The most accurate way to measure a regular rhythm is to count the number of small boxes between two R waves. That number is divided into 1500 to calculate bpm. Remember: 60 sec/min divided by 0.04 sec/small box =1500 small boxes/min.

Examples:
If there are three small boxes between two R waves: 1500/3 = 500 bpm.
If there are five small boxes between two R waves: 1500/5 = 300 bpm.

Methods 1 and 2 for Calculating Heart Rate

Number of Large Boxes	Rate/Min	Number of Small Boxes	Rate/Min
1	300	2	750
2	150	3	500
3	100	4	375
4	75	5	300
5	60	6	250
6	50	7	214
7	43	8	186
8	38	9	167
9	33	10	150
10	30	11	136
11	27	12	125
12	25	13	115
13	23	14	107
14	21	15	100
15	20	16	94

♥ **Clinical Tip:** Approximate rate/min is rounded to the next-highest number.

Notes:

Method 3: Six-Second ECG Rhythm Strip

The best method for measuring irregular heart rates with varying R-R intervals is to count the number of R waves in a 6-sec strip (including extra beats such as PVCs, PACs, and PJCs) and multiply by 10. This gives the average number of beats per minute.

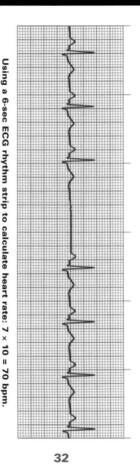

Using a 6-sec ECG rhythm strip to calculate heart rate: 7 × 10 = 70 bpm.

● **Clinical Tip:** If a rhythm is extremely irregular, it is best to count the number of R-R intervals per 60 sec (1 min).

ECG Interpretation

Analyzing a Rhythm	
Component	**Characteristic**
Rate	The bpm is commonly the ventricular rate. If atrial and ventricular rates differ, as in a 3rd-degree block, measure both rates. Normal: 60–100 bpm Slow (bradycardia): <60 bpm Fast (tachycardia): >100 bpm
Regularity	Measure R-R intervals and P-P intervals. Regular: Intervals consistent Regularly irregular: Repeating pattern Irregular: No pattern
P Waves	If present: Same in size, shape, position? Does each QRS have a P wave? Normal: Upright (positive) and uniform Inverted: Negative Notched: P' None: Rhythm is junctional or ventricular.
PR Interval	Constant: Intervals are the same Variable: Intervals differ Normal: 0.12–0.20 sec and constant
QRS Interval	Normal: 0.06–0.10 sec Wide: >0.10 sec None: Absent
QT Interval	Beginning of QRS complex to end of T wave Varies with HR Normal: Less than half the RR interval
QTc Interval	The QTc interval is the QT interval corrected for the heart rate. Formula for calculating QTc: QTc = QT divided by the square root of the R to R interval Normal corrected QTc should be < 0.44 seconds.
Dropped beats	Occur in AV blocks Occur in sinus arrest

Analyzing a Rhythm—cont'd.	
Component	**Characteristic**
Pause	Compensatory: Complete pause following a premature atrial contraction (PAC), premature junctional contraction (PJC), or premature ventricular contraction (PVC)
	Noncompensatory: Incomplete pause following a PAC, PJC, or PVC
QRS Complex grouping	Bigeminy: Repeating pattern of normal complex followed by a premature complex
	Trigeminy: Repeating pattern of 2 normal complexes followed by a premature complex
	Quadrigeminy: Repeating pattern of 3 normal complexes followed by a premature complex
	Couplet: 2 Consecutive premature complexes
	Triplet: 3 Consecutive premature complexes

Classification of Arrhythmias	
Heart Rate	**Classification**
Slow	Bradyarrhythmia
Fast	Tachyarrhythmia
Absent	Pulseless arrest

Normal Heart Rate (bpm)			
Age	**Awake Rate**	**Mean**	**Sleeping Rate**
Newborn to 3 months	85–205	140	80–160
3 months to 2 years	100–190	130	75–160
2 to 10 years	60–140	80	60–90
>10 years	60–100	75	50–90

Sinoatrial (SA) Node Arrhythmias

- Upright P waves all look similar. **Note: All ECG strips in Tab 2 were recorded in lead II.**
- PR intervals and QRS complexes are of normal duration.

Normal Sinus Rhythm (NSR)

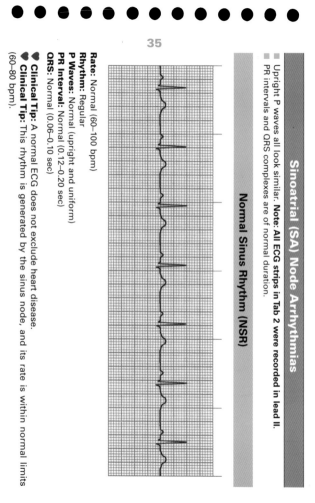

Rate: Normal (60–100 bpm)

Rhythm: Regular

P Waves: Normal (upright and uniform)

PR Interval: Normal (0.12–0.20 sec)

QRS: Normal (0.06–0.10 sec)

♥ **Clinical Tip:** A normal ECG does not exclude heart disease.

♥ **Clinical Tip:** This rhythm is generated by the sinus node, and its rate is within normal limits (60–80 bpm).

Sinus Bradycardia

■ The SA node discharges more slowly than in NSR.

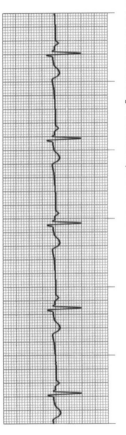

Rate: Slow (<60 bpm)

Rhythm: Regular

P Waves: Normal (upright and uniform)

PR Interval: Normal (0.12–0.20 sec)

QRS: Normal (0.06—0.10 sec)

♥ **Clinical Tip:** Sinus bradycardia is normal in athletes and during sleep. In acute MI, it may be protective and beneficial, or the slow rate may compromise cardiac output. Certain medications, such as beta blockers, may also cause sinus bradycardia. Sinus bradycardia may also be caused by vagal stimulation, such as gagging, straining, and endotracheal suctioning, and by chronic ischemic heart disease, sick sinus syndrome, hypothyroidism, and increased intracranial pressure.

Sinus Tachycardia

- The SA node discharges more frequently than in NSR.

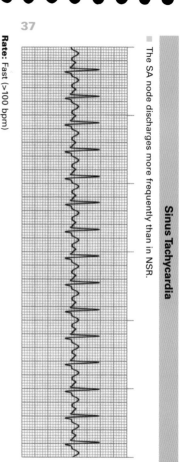

Rate: Fast (>100 bpm)

Rhythm: Regular

P Waves: Normal (upright and uniform)

PR Interval: Normal (0.12–0.20 sec)

QRS: Normal (0.06–0.10 sec)

♥ **Clinical Tip:** Sinus tachycardia may be caused by conditions such as fear, pain, exercise, anxiety, or fever. But it can also have a more significant pathological cause such as hypoxemia; hypovolemia and dehydration; cardiac failure or recent MI; CHF; beta blocker withdrawal; hyperthyroidism; or nicotine, alcohol, caffeine, and alcohol withdrawal.

Sinus Arrhythmia

- The SA node discharges irregularly.
- The R-R interval is irregular.

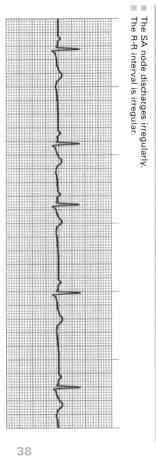

Rate: Usually normal (60–100 bpm); frequently increases with inspiration and decreases with expiration; may be <60 bpm

Rhythm: Irregular; varies with respiration; difference between shortest RR and longest RR intervals is >0.12 sec

P Waves: Normal (upright and uniform)

PR Interval: Normal (0.12–0.20 sec)

QRS: Normal (0.06–0.10 sec)

♥ **Clinical Tip:** The pacing rate of the SA node varies with respiration, especially in children and elderly people.

Sinus Pause (Sinus Arrest)

- The SA node fails to discharge and then resumes.
- Electrical activity resumes either when the SA node resets itself or when a slower latent pacemaker begins to discharge.
- The pause (arrest) time interval is not a multiple of the normal PP interval.

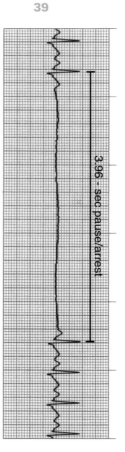

3.96 - sec pause/arrest

Rate: Normal to slow; determined by duration and frequency of sinus pause (arrest)

Rhythm: Irregular whenever a pause (arrest) occurs

P Waves: Normal (upright and uniform) except in areas of pause (arrest)

PR Interval: Normal (0.12–0.20 sec)

QRS: Normal (0.06–0.10 sec)

❤ **Clinical Tip:** Cardiac output may decrease, causing syncope or dizziness.

Sinoatrial (SA) Block

- The block occurs in some multiple of the PP interval.
- After the dropped beat, cycles continue on time.

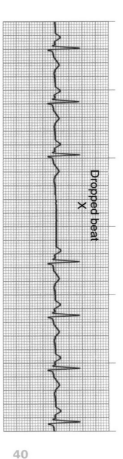

Dropped beat
X

Rate: Normal to slow; determined by duration and frequency of SA block

Rhythm: Irregular whenever an SA block occurs

P Waves: Normal (upright and uniform) except in areas of dropped beats

PR Interval: Normal (0.12–0.20 sec)

QRS: Normal (0.06–0.10 sec)

♥ **Clinical Tip:** Cardiac output may decrease, causing syncope or dizziness.

Atrial Arrhythmias

- P waves differ in appearance from sinus P waves.
- QRS complexes are of normal duration if no ventricular conduction disturbances are present.

Wandering Atrial Pacemaker (WAP)

Pacemaker site transfers from the SA node to other latent pacemaker sites in the atria and the AV junction and then moves back to the SA node.

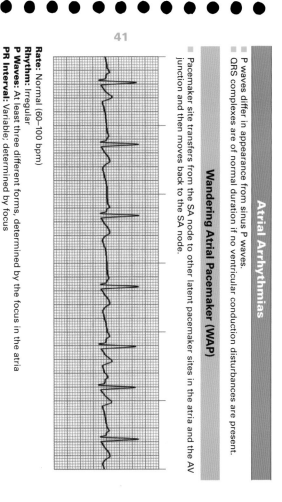

Rate: Normal (60–100 bpm)

Rhythm: Irregular

P Waves: At least three different forms, determined by the focus in the atria

PR Interval: Variable; determined by focus

QRS: Normal (0.06–0.10 sec)

❤ **Clinical Tip:** WAP may occur in normal hearts as a result of fluctuations in vagal tone.

Multifocal Atrial Tachycardia (MAT)

■ This form of WAP is associated with a ventricular response >100 bpm.
■ MAT may be confused with atrial fibrillation (A-fib); however, MAT has a visible P wave.

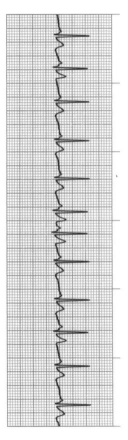

Rate: Fast (>100 bpm)

Rhythm: Irregular

P Wave: At least three different forms, determined by the focus in the atria

PR Interval: Variable; determined by focus

QRS: Normal (0.06–0.10 sec)

♥ **Clinical Tip:** MAT is commonly seen in patients with chronic obstructive pulmonary disease (COPD) but may also occur in those with an acute MI.

Premature Atrial Contraction (PAC)

- A single contraction occurs earlier than the next expected sinus contraction.
- After the PAC, sinus rhythm usually resumes.

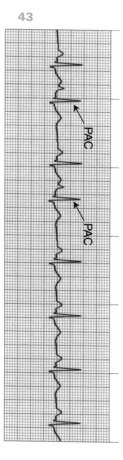

PAC

PAC

Rate: Depends on rate of underlying rhythm

Rhythm: Irregular whenever a PAC occurs

P Waves: Present; in the PAC, may have a different shape

PR Interval: Varies in the PAC; otherwise normal (0.12–0.20 sec)

QRS: Normal (0.06–0.10 sec)

♥ **Clinical Tip:** In patients with heart disease, frequent PACs may precede paroxysmal supraventricular tachycardia (PSVT), atrial fibrillation (A-fib), or atrial flutter (A-flutter).

Atrial Tachycardia

- A rapid atrial rate overrides the SA node and becomes the dominant pacemaker.
- Some ST segment and T wave abnormalities may be present.

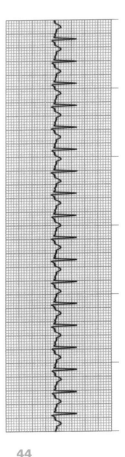

Rate: 150–250 bpm

Rhythm: Regular

P Waves: Normal (upright and uniform) but differ in shape from sinus P waves

PR Interval: May be short (<0.12 sec) in rapid rates

QRS: Normal (0.06–0.10 sec) but can be aberrant at times

Supraventricular Tachycardia (SVT)

■ This arrhythmia has such a fast rate that the P waves may not be seen.

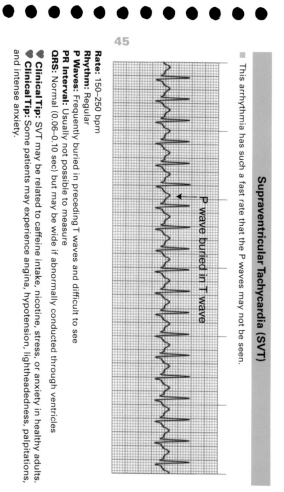

P wave buried in T wave

Rate: 150–250 bpm

Rhythm: Regular

P Waves: Frequently buried in preceding T waves and difficult to see

PR Interval: Usually not possible to measure

QRS: Normal (0.06–0.10 sec) but may be wide if abnormally conducted through ventricles

◆◆ **Clinical Tip:** SVT may be related to caffeine intake, nicotine, stress, or anxiety in healthy adults.

◆◆ **Clinical Tip:** Some patients may experience angina, hypotension, lightheadedness, palpitations, and intense anxiety.

Paroxysmal Supraventricular Tachycardia (PSVT)

▪ PSVT is a rapid rhythm that starts and stops suddenly.
▪ For accurate interpretation, the beginning or end of the PSVT must be seen.
▪ PSVT is sometimes called paroxysmal atrial tachycardia (PAT).

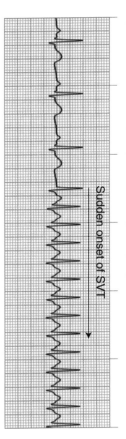

Sudden onset of SVT

Rate: 150–250 bpm

Rhythm: Irregular

P Waves: Frequently buried in preceding T waves and difficult to see

PR Interval: Usually not possible to measure

QRS: Normal (0.06–0.10 sec) but may be wide if abnormally conducted through ventricles

♥ **Clinical Tip:** The patient may feel palpitations, dizziness, lightheadedness, or anxiety.

Atrial Flutter (A-flutter)

- AV node conducts impulses to the ventricles at a ratio of 2:1, 3:1, 4:1, or greater (rarely 1:1).
- The degree of AV block may be consistent or variable.

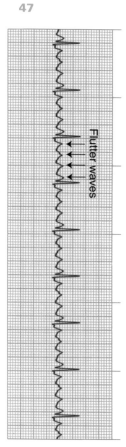

Flutter waves

Rate: Atrial: 250–350 bpm; ventricular: variable

Rhythm: Atrial: regular; ventricular: variable

P Waves: Flutter waves have a saw-toothed appearance; some may be buried in the QRS and not visible

PR Interval: Variable

QRS: Usually normal (0.06–0.10 sec), but may appear widened if flutter waves are buried in QRS

◆ **Clinical Tip:** A-flutter may be the first indication of cardiac disease.

◆ **Clinical Tip:** Signs and symptoms depend on ventricular response rate.

Atrial Fibrillation (A-fib)

- Rapid, erratic electrical discharge comes from multiple atrial ectopic foci.
- No organized atrial depolarization is detectable.

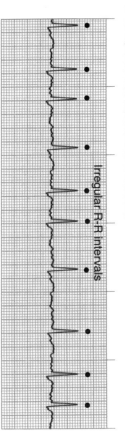

Irregular R-R intervals

Rate: Atrial: ≧350 bpm; ventricular: variable
Rhythm: Irregular
P Waves: No true P waves; chaotic atrial activity
PR Interval: None
QRS: Normal (0.06–0.10 sec)

❤❤ **Clinical Tip:** A-fib is usually a chronic arrhythmia associated with underlying heart disease.
❤❤ **Clinical Tip:** Signs and symptoms depend on ventricular response rate.

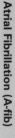

Wolff-Parkinson-White (WPW) Syndrome

- In WPW, an accessory conduction pathway is present between the atria and the ventricles.
- Electrical impulses are rapidly conducted to the ventricles.
- These rapid impulses slur the initial portion of the QRS; the slurred effect is called a delta wave.

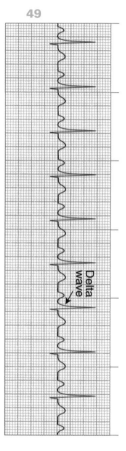

Delta wave

Rate: Depends on rate of underlying rhythm

Rhythm: Regular unless associated with A-fib

P Waves: Normal (upright and uniform) unless A-fib is present

PR Interval: Short (<0.12 sec) if P wave is present

QRS: Wide (>0.10 sec); delta wave present

♥ **Clinical Tip:** WPW is associated with narrow-complex tachycardias, including A-flutter and A-fib.

Junctional Arrhythmias

- The atria and SA node do not perform their normal pacemaking functions.
- A junctional escape rhythm begins.

Junctional Rhythm

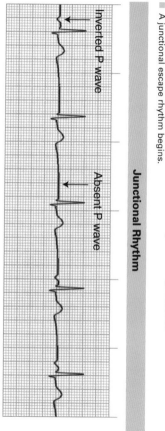

Inverted P wave

Absent P wave

Rate: 40–60 bpm

Rhythm: Regular

P Waves: Absent, inverted, buried, or retrograde

PR Interval: None, short, or retrograde

QRS: Normal (0.06–0.10 sec)

♥ **Clinical Tip:** Sinus node disease that causes inappropriate slowing of the sinus node may exacerbate this rhythm. Young, healthy adults, especially those with increased vagal tone during sleep, often have periods of junctional rhythm that is completely benign, not requiring intervention.

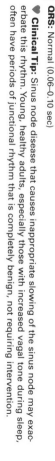

Accelerated Junctional Rhythm

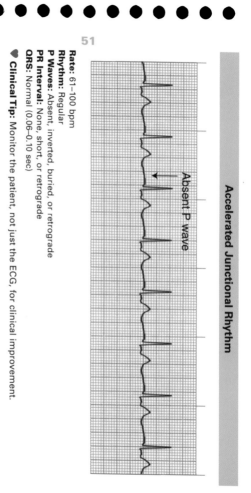

Absent P wave

Rate: 61–100 bpm

Rhythm: Regular

P Waves: Absent, inverted, buried, or retrograde

PR Interval: None, short, or retrograde

QRS: Normal (0.06–0.10 sec)

♥ **Clinical Tip:** Monitor the patient, not just the ECG, for clinical improvement.

Junctional Tachycardia

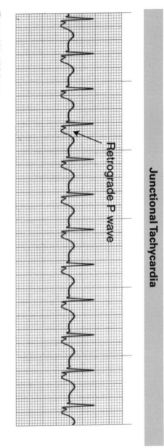

Retrograde P wave

Rate: 101–180 bpm

Rhythm: Regular

P Waves: Absent, inverted, buried, or retrograde

PR Interval: None, short, or retrograde

QRS: Normal (0.06–0.10 sec)

● **Clinical Tip:** Signs and symptoms of decreased cardiac output may be seen in response to the rapid rate.

Junctional Escape Beat

■ An escape complex comes later than the next expected sinus complex.

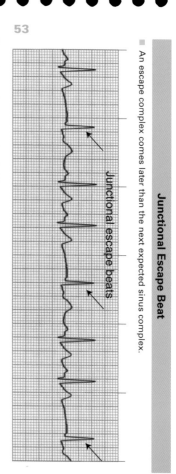

Junctional escape beats

Rate: Depends on rate of underlying rhythm
Rhythm: Irregular whenever an escape beat occurs
P Waves: None, inverted, buried, or retrograde in the escape beat
PR Interval: None, short, or retrograde
QRS: Normal (0.06–0.10 sec)

53

Premature Junctional Contraction (PJC)

■ Enhanced automaticity in the AV junction produces PJCs.

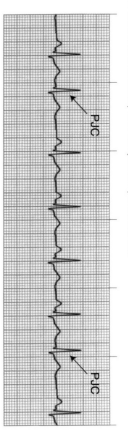

Rate: Depends on rate of underlying rhythm

Rhythm: Irregular whenever a PJC occurs

P Waves: Absent, inverted, buried, or retrograde in the PJC

PR Interval: None, short, or retrograde

QRS: Normal (0.06–0.10 sec)

❤ **Clinical Tip:** Before deciding whether isolated PJCs are insignificant, consider the cause.

Ventricular Arrhythmias

■ In all ventricular rhythms, the QRS complex is >0.10 sec. P Waves are absent or, if visible, have no consistent relationship to the QRS complex.

Idioventricular Rhythm

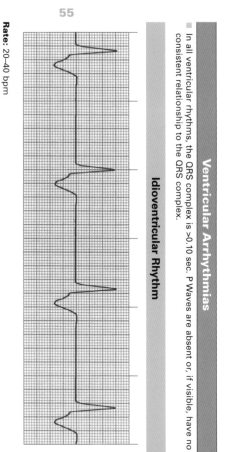

Rate: 20–40 bpm
Rhythm: Regular
P Waves: None
PR Interval: None
QRS: Wide (>0.10 sec), bizarre appearance

♥ **Clinical Tip:** Diminished cardiac output is expected because of the slow heart rate. An idioventricular rhythm may be called an agonal rhythm when the heart rate drops below 20 bpm. An agonal rhythm is generally terminal and is usually the last rhythm before asystole.

Accelerated Idioventricular Rhythm

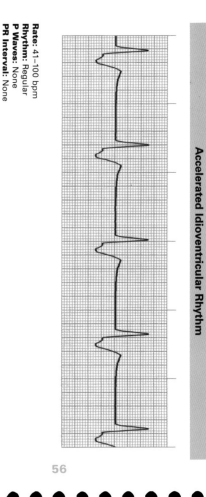

Rate: 41–100 bpm
Rhythm: Regular
P Waves: None
PR Interval: None
QRS: Wide (>0.10 sec), bizarre appearance

♥ **ClinicalTip:** Idioventricular rhythms appear when supraventricular pacing sites are depressed or absent. Diminished cardiac output is expected if the heart rate is slow.

Premature Ventricular Contraction (PVC)

PVCs result from an irritable ventricular focus.

PVCs may be uniform (same form) or multiform (different forms).

Usually a PVC is followed by a full compensatory pause because the sinus node timing is not interrupted. In contrast, a PVC may be followed by a noncompensatory pause if the PVC enters the sinus node and resets its timing, enabling the following sinus P wave to appear earlier than expected.

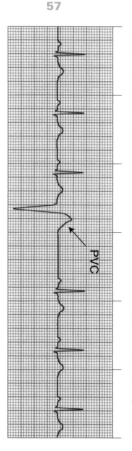

PVC

Rate: Depends on rate of underlying rhythm

Rhythm: Irregular whenever a PVC occurs

P Waves: None associated with the PVC

PR Interval: None associated with the PVC

QRS: Wide (>0.10 sec), bizarre appearance

● **Clinical Tip:** Patients may sense PVCs as skipped beats. Because the ventricles are only partially filled, the PVC frequently does not generate a pulse.

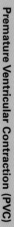

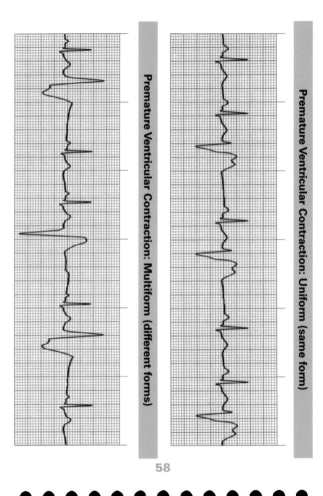

Premature Ventricular Contraction: Uniform (same form)

Premature Ventricular Contraction: Multiform (different forms)

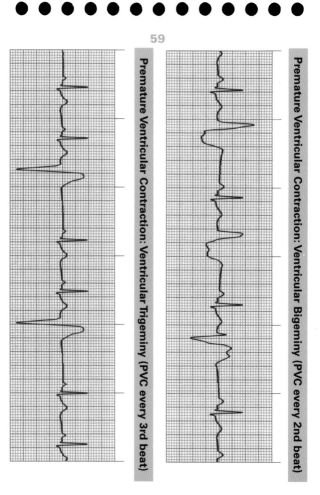

Premature Ventricular Contraction: Ventricular Trigeminy (PVC every 3rd beat)

Premature Ventricular Contraction: Ventricular Bigeminy (PVC every 2nd beat)

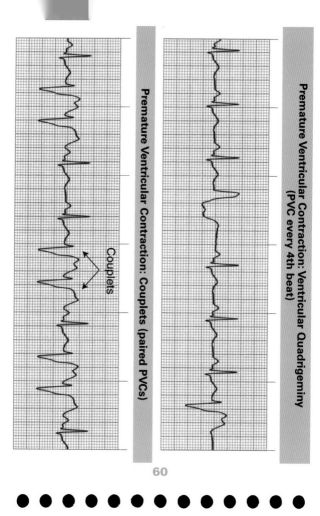

Premature Ventricular Contraction: Couplets (paired PVCs)

Couplets

Premature Ventricular Contraction: Ventricular Quadrigeminy (PVC every 4th beat)

60

Premature Ventricular Contraction: R-on-T Phenomenon

- The PVCs occur so early that they fall on the T wave of the preceding beat.
- These PVCs occur during the refractory period of the ventricles, a vulnerable period because the cardiac cells have not fully repolarized.

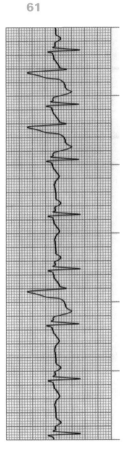
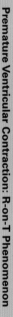

Rate: Depends on rate of underlying rhythm

Rhythm: Irregular whenever a PVC occurs

P Waves: None associated with the PVC

PR Interval: None associated with the PVC

QRS: Wide (>0.10 sec), bizarre appearance

● **Clinical Tip:** In acute ischemia, R-on-T phenomenon may be especially dangerous because the ventricles may be more vulnerable to ventricular tachycardia (VT), ventricular fibrillation (VF), or torsades de pointes.

Premature Contraction: Interpolated PVC

- The PVC occurs between two regular complexes; it may appear sandwiched between two normal beats.
- An interpolated PVC does not interfere with the normal cardiac cycle.

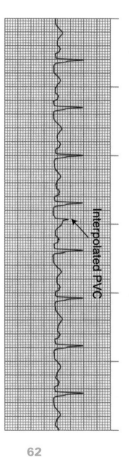

Interpolated PVC

Rate: Depends on rate of underlying rhythm
Rhythm: Irregular whenever a PVC occurs
P Waves: None associated with the PVC
PR Interval: None associated with the PVC
QRS: Wide (>0.10 sec), bizarre appearance

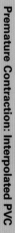

Ventricular Tachycardia (VT): Monomorphic

- In monomorphic VT, QRS complexes have the same shape and amplitude.

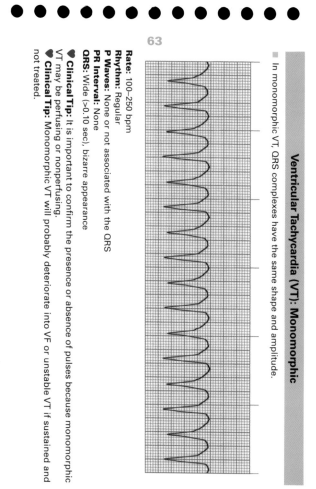

Rate: 100–250 bpm

Rhythm: Regular

P Waves: None or not associated with the QRS

PR Interval: None

QRS: Wide (>0.10 sec), bizarre appearance

♥ **Clinical Tip:** It is important to confirm the presence or absence of pulses because monomorphic VT may be perfusing or nonperfusing.

♥ **Clinical Tip:** Monomorphic VT will probably deteriorate into VF or unstable VT if sustained and not treated.

Ventricular Tachycardia (VT): Polymorphic

- In polymorphic VT, QRS complexes vary in shape and amplitude.
- The QT interval is normal or long.

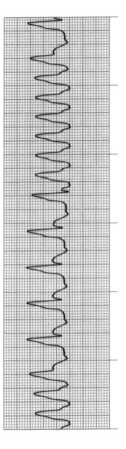

Rate: 100–250 bpm

Rhythm: Regular or irregular

P Waves: None or not associated with the QRS

PR Interval: None

QRS: Wide (>0.10 sec), bizarre appearance

● **Clinical Tip:** It is important to determine whether pulses are present because polymorphic VT may be perfusing or nonperfusing.

◆ **Clinical Tip:** Consider electrolyte abnormalities as a possible cause.

Torsade de Pointes

■ The QRS reverses polarity, and the strip shows a spindle effect.
■ This rhythm is an unusual variant of polymorphic VT with long QT intervals.
■ In French, the term means "twisting of points."

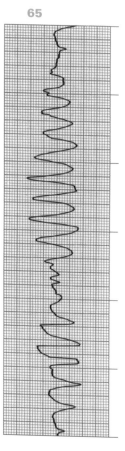
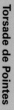

Rate: 200–250 bpm
Rhythm: Irregular
P Waves: None
PR Interval: None
QRS: Wide (>0.10 sec), bizarre appearance

♥ **Clinical Tip:** Torsade de pointes may deteriorate to VF or asystole.
♥ **Clinical Tip:** Frequent causes are drugs that prolong the QT interval, electrolyte abnormalities such as hypomagnesemia, or the R-on-T phenomenon.

Ventricular Fibrillation (VF)

■ Chaotic electrical activity occurs with no ventricular depolarization or contraction.
■ The amplitude and frequency of the fibrillatory activity can define the type of fibrillation as coarse, medium, or fine. Small baseline undulations are considered fine; large ones are coarse.

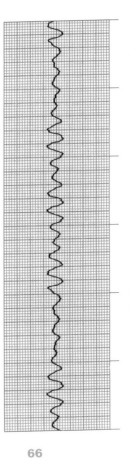

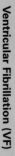

Rate: Indeterminate
Rhythm: Chaotic
P Waves: None
PR Interval: None
QRS: None

♥ **Clinical Tip:** There is no pulse or cardiac output. Rapid intervention is critical. The longer the delay, the less the chance for conversion.

Pulseless Electrical Activity (PEA)

- The monitor shows an identifiable electrical rhythm, but no pulse is detected.
- The rhythm may be sinus, atrial, junctional, or ventricular.
- PEA is also called electromechanical dissociation (EMD).

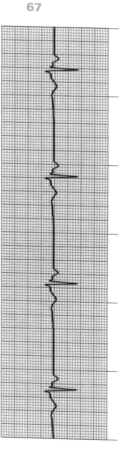

Rate: Reflects underlying rhythm

Rhythm: Reflects underlying rhythm

P Waves: Reflect underlying rhythm

PR Interval: Reflects underlying rhythm

QRS: Reflects underlying rhythm

♥ **Clinical Tip:** Potential causes of PEA are trauma, tension pneumothorax, thrombosis (pulmonary or coronary), cardiac tamponade, toxins, hypokalemia or hyperkalemia, hypovolemia, hypoxia, hypoglycemia, hypothermia, and hydrogen ion (acidosis).

Asystole

■ Electrical activity in the ventricles is completely absent.

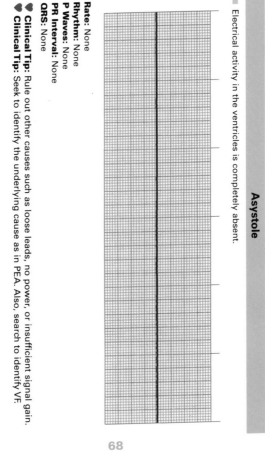

Rate: None
Rhythm: None
P Waves: None
PR Interval: None
QRS: None

♦♦ **Clinical Tip:** Rule out other causes such as loose leads, no power, or insufficient signal gain.
◆◆ **Clinical Tip:** Seek to identify the underlying cause as in PEA. Also, search to identify VF.

Atrioventricular (AV) Blocks

■ AV blocks are divided into three categories: first, second, and third degree.

First-Degree AV Block

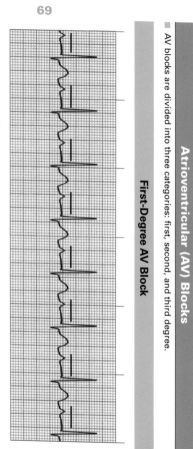

Rate: Depends on rate of underlying rhythm

Rhythm: Regular

P Waves: Normal (upright and uniform)

PR Interval: Prolonged (>0.20 sec)

QRS: Normal (0.06–0.10 sec)

♥ **Clinical Tip:** Usually a first-degree AV block is benign, but if associated with an acute MI, it may lead to further AV defects.

♥ **Clinical Tip:** Often AV block is caused by medications that prolong AV conduction; these include digoxin, calcium channel blockers, and beta blockers.

Second-Degree AV Block—Type I (Mobitz I or Wenckebach)

■ PR intervals become progressively longer until one P wave is totally blocked and produces no QRS complex. After a pause, during which the AV node recovers, this cycle is repeated.

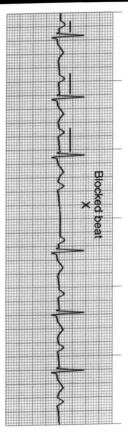

Blocked beat
X

Rate: Depends on rate of underlying rhythm

Rhythm: Atrial: regular; ventricular: irregular

P Waves: Normal (upright and uniform); more P waves than QRS complexes

PR Interval: Progressively longer until one P wave is blocked and a QRS is dropped

QRS: Normal (0.06–0.10 sec)

● **Clinical Tip:** This rhythm may be caused by medication such as beta blockers, digoxin, and calcium channel blockers. Ischemia involving the right coronary artery is another cause.

Second-Degree AV Block—Type II (Mobitz II)

- Conduction ratio (P waves to QRS complexes) is commonly 2:1, 3:1, or 4:1, or variable.
- QRS complexes are usually wide because this block usually involves both bundle branches.

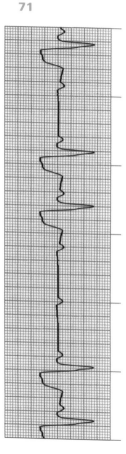

Rate: Atrial: usually 60–100 bpm; ventricular: slower than atrial rate

Rhythm: Atrial: regular; ventricular: regular or irregular

P Waves: Normal (upright and uniform); more P waves than QRS complexes

PR Interval: Normal or prolonged but constant

QRS: May be normal, but usually wide (>0.10 sec) if the bundle branches are involved

💗 **Clinical Tip:** Resulting bradycardia can compromise cardiac output and lead to complete AV block. This rhythm often occurs with cardiac ischemia or an MI.

Third-Degree AV Block

- Conduction between atria and ventricles is totally absent because of complete electrical block at or below the AV node. This is known as AV dissociation.
- "Complete heart block" is another name for this rhythm.

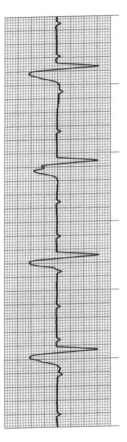

Rate: Atrial: 60–100 bpm; ventricular: 40–60 bpm if escape focus is junctional, <40 bpm if escape focus is ventricular

Rhythm: Usually regular, but atria and ventricles act independently

P Waves: Normal (upright and uniform); may be superimposed on QRS complexes or T waves

PR Interval: Varies greatly

QRS: Normal if ventricles are activated by junctional escape focus; wide if escape focus is ventricular

● **Clinical Tip:** Third-degree AV block may be associated with ischemia involving the left coronary arteries.

Bundle Branch Block (BBB)

■ Either the left or the right ventricle may depolarize late, creating a "wide" or "notched" QRS complex.

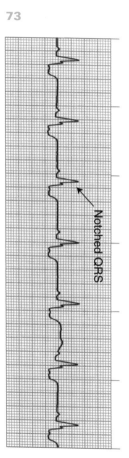

Notched QRS

Rate: Depends on rate of underlying rhythm

Rhythm: Regular

P Waves: Normal (upright and uniform)

PR Interval: Normal (0.12–0.20 sec)

QRS: Wide (>0.10 sec) with a notched appearance

♥ **Clinical Tip:** Bundle branch block commonly occurs in coronary artery disease.

Artificial Cardiac Pacemakers

- Artificial pacemakers electronically stimulate the heart in place of the heart's own pacemaker.
- Pacemakers may be preset to stimulate the heart's activity continuously or intermittently.

Temporary Pacemaker

- Paces the heart through epicardial, transvenous, or transcutaneous routes. The pulse generator is located externally.

Permanent Pacemaker

- Its circuitry sealed in an airtight case, the pacemaker is implanted in the body. It uses sensing and pacing device leads.

Single-Chamber Pacemaker

- One lead is placed in the heart and paces a single heart chamber (either atrium or ventricle).

Dual-Chamber Pacemaker

- One lead is placed in the right atrium and the other in the right ventricle. The atrial electrode generates a spike that should be followed by a P wave, and the ventricular electrode generates a spike followed by a wide QRS complex.

74

Pacemaker Modes

- Fixed rate (asynchronous): Discharges at a preset rate (usually 70–80 bpm) regardless of the patient's own electrical activity.
- Demand (synchronous): Discharges only when the patient's heart rate drops below the pacemaker's preset (base) rate.

♥ **Clinical Tip:** Patients with pacemakers may receive defibrillation, but avoid placing the defibrillator paddles or pads closer than 5 inches to the pacemaker battery pack.

Arttificial Cardiac Pacemakers

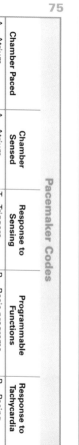

Pacemaker Codes

Chamber Paced	Chamber Sensed	Response to Sensing	Programmable Functions	Response to Tachycardia
A = Atrium	A = Atrium	T = Triggers pacing	P = Basic programs (rate and output)	P = Pacing
V = Ventricle	V = Ventricle	I = Inhibits pacing	M = Multiple programs	S = Shock
D = Dual (atrium and ventricle)	D = Dual (atrium and ventricle)	D = Dual (triggers and inhibits)	C = Communication (i.e., telemetry)	D = Dual (pace and shock)
O = None	O = None	O = None	R = Rate response	O = None
			O = None	

Artificial Pacemaker Rhythm

Rate	Varies according to preset pacemaker rate.
Rhythm	Regular for asynchronous pacemaker; irregular for demand pacemaker unless 100% paced with no intrinsic beats.
P Waves	None produced by ventricular pacemaker. Sinus P waves may be seen but are unrelated to QRS. Atrial or dual-chamber pacemaker should have P waves following each atrial spike.
PR Interval	None for ventricular pacer. Atrial or dual-chamber pacemaker produces constant PR intervals.
QRS	Wide (>0.10 sec) following each ventricular spike in a pacemaker rhythm. The patient's own electrical activity may generate a QRS complex that looks different from the paced QRSs. If atrially paced only, the QRS may be within normal limits.

● **Clinical Tip:** Once an impulse is generated by the pacemaker, it appears as a spike, either above or below the baseline (isoelectric line), on the ECG. The spike indicates that the pacemaker has fired.
● **Clinical Tip:** A pacemaker is in capture when a spike produces an ECG wave or complex.

76

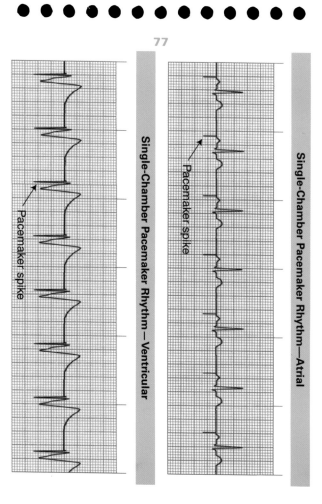

Single-Chamber Pacemaker Rhythm—Ventricular

Pacemaker spike

Single-Chamber Pacemaker Rhythm—Atrial

Pacemaker spike

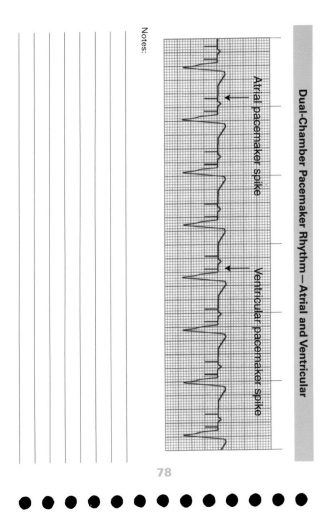

Dual-Chamber Pacemaker Rhythm—Atrial and Ventricular

Atrial pacemaker spike

Ventricular pacemaker spike

Notes:

Pacemaker Malfunctions

Malfunction	Reason
Failure to pace	Pacemaker spikes are absent. The cause may be a dead battery, a disruption in the connecting wires, or improper programming.
Failure to capture	Pacemaker spikes are present, but no P wave or QRS follows the spike. Turning up the pacemaker's voltage often corrects this problem. Lead wires should also be checked—a dislodged or broken lead wire may not deliver the needed energy.
Failure to sense	The pacemaker fires because it fails to detect the heart's intrinsic beats, resulting in abnormal complexes. The cause may be a dead battery, decrease of P wave or QRS voltage, or damage to a pacing lead wire. One serious potential consequence may be an R-on-T phenomenon.
Oversensing	The pacemaker may be too sensitive and misinterpret muscle movement or other events in the cardiac cycle as depolarization. This error resets the pacemaker inappropriately, increasing the amount of time before the next discharge.

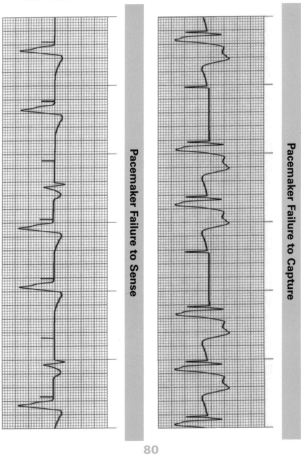

Pacemaker Failure to Sense

Pacemaker Failure to Capture

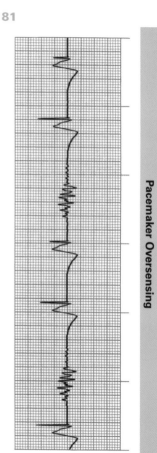

Pacemaker Oversensing

Artifacts are ECG deflections caused by influences other than the heart's electrical activity.

Loose Electrodes

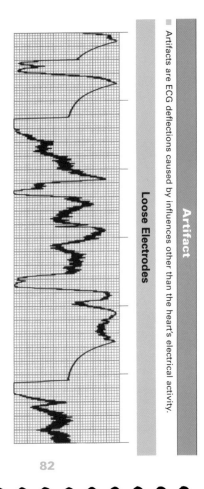

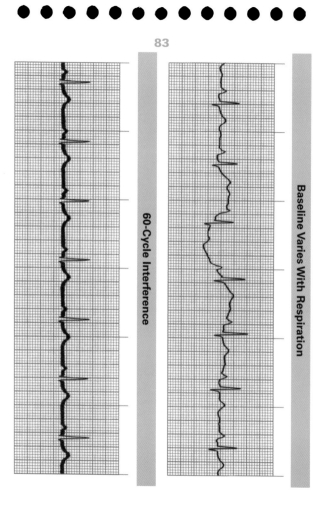

60-Cycle Interference

Baseline Varies With Respiration

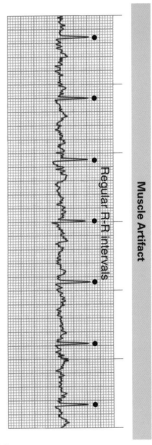

Muscle Artifact

Regular R-R intervals

❤ **Clinical Tip:** Never confuse muscle artifact with A-fib if the rhythm is regular.

84

Notes:

The 12-Lead ECG

A standard 12-lead ECG provides views of the heart from 12 different angles. This diagnostic test helps to identify pathological conditions, especially bundle branch blocks and T wave changes associated with ischemia, injury, and infarction. The 12-lead ECG also uses ST segment analysis to pinpoint the specific location of an MI.

The 12-lead ECG is the type most commonly used in clinical settings. The following list highlights some of its important aspects:

- The 12-lead ECG consists of the six limb leads—I, II, III, aVR, aVL, and aVF—and the six chest leads—V_1, V_2, V_3, V_4, V_5, and V_6.
- The limb leads record electrical activity in the heart's frontal plane. This view shows the middle of the heart from top to bottom. Electrical activity is recorded from the anterior to posterior axis.
- The chest leads record electrical activity in the heart's horizontal plane. This transverse view shows the middle of the heart from left to right, dividing it into upper and lower portions. Electrical activity is recorded from either a superior or an inferior approach.
- Measurements are central to 12-lead ECG analysis. The height and depth of waves can offer important diagnostic information in certain conditions, including MI and ventricular hypertrophy.
- The direction of ventricular depolarization is an important factor in determining the axis of the heart.
- In an MI, multiple leads are necessary to recognize its presence and determine its location. If large areas of the heart are affected, the patient can develop cardiogenic shock and fatal arrhythmias.
- ECG signs of an MI are best seen in the reciprocal, or reflecting, leads—those facing the affected surface of the heart. Reciprocal leads are in the same plane but opposite the area of infarction; they show a mirror image of the electrical complex.
- Prehospital EMS systems may use 12-lead ECGs to discover signs of acute MI, such as ST segment elevation, in preparation for in-hospital administration of thrombolytic drugs.
- After a 12-lead ECG is performed, a 15-lead, or right-sided, ECG may be used for an even more comprehensive view if the right ventricle or the posterior portion of the heart appears to be affected.

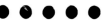

R Wave Progression

- Normal ventricular depolarization in the heart progresses from right to left and from front to back.
- In a normal heart, the R wave becomes taller and the S wave smaller as electrical activity crosses the heart from right to left. This phenomenon is called R wave progression and is noted on the chest leads.
- Alteration in the normal R wave progression may be seen in left ventricular hypertrophy, COPD, left bundle branch block, or anteroseptal MI.

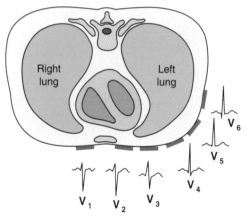

Normal R wave progression in chest leads V₁–V₆

Electrical Axis Deviation

- The electrical axis is the sum total of all electrical currents generated by the ventricular myocardium during depolarization.
- Analysis of the axis may help to determine the location and extent of cardiac injury, such as ventricular hypertrophy, bundle branch block, or changes in the position of the heart in the chest (e.g., from pregnancy or ascites).
- The direction of the QRS complex in leads I and aVF determines the axis quadrant in relation to the heart.

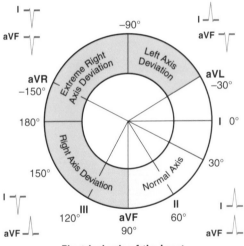

Electrical axis of the heart

💙 **Clinical Tip:** Extreme right axis deviation is also called indeterminate, "no man's land," and "northwest."

Ischemia, Injury, and Infarction in Relation to the Heart

Ischemia, injury, and infarction of cardiac tissue are the three stages resulting from complete blockage in a coronary artery. The location of the MI is critical in determining the most appropriate treatment and predicting probable complications. Each coronary artery delivers blood to specific areas of the heart. Blockages at different sites can damage various parts of the heart. Characteristic ECG changes occur in different leads with each type of MI and can be correlated to the blockages.

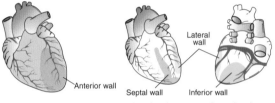

Anterior wall

Anterior view

Septal wall   Inferior wall   Lateral wall

Anterior view   Posterior view

Location of MI by ECG Leads

I lateral	aVR	V$_1$ septal	V$_4$ anterior
II inferior	aVL lateral	V$_2$ septal	V$_5$ lateral
III inferior	aVF inferior	V$_3$ anterior	V$_6$ lateral

♥ **Clinical Tip:** Lead aVR may not show any change in an MI.
♥ **Clinical Tip:** An MI may not be limited to just one region of the heart. For example, if there are changes in leads V$_3$ and V$_4$ (anterior) and leads I, aVL, V$_5$, and V$_6$ (lateral), the MI is called an anterolateral infarction.

Progression of an Acute Myocardial Infarction

An acute MI is a continuum that extends from the normal state to a full infarction:

- Ischemia—Lack of oxygen to the cardiac tissue, represented by ST segment depression, T wave inversion, or both
- Injury—Arterial occlusion with ischemia, represented by ST segment elevation
- Infarction—Death of tissue, represented by a pathological Q wave

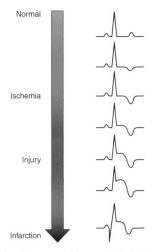

♥ **Clinical Tip:** After the acute MI has ended, the ST segment returns to baseline and the T wave becomes upright, but the Q wave remains abnormal because of scar formation.

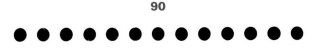

ST Segment Elevation and Depression

- A normal ST segment represents early ventricular repolarization.
- Displacement of the ST segment can be caused by the following various conditions:

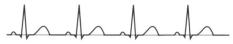

ST segment is at baseline.

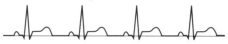

ST segment is elevated.

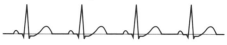

ST segment is depressed.

Primary Causes of ST Segment Elevation

- ST segment elevation exceeding 1 mm in the limb leads and 2 mm in the chest leads indicates an evolving acute MI until there is proof to the contrary. Other primary causes of ST segment elevation are:
  - Early repolarization (normal variant in young adults)
  - Pericarditis, ventricular aneurysm
  - Pulmonary embolism, intracranial hemorrhage

Primary Causes of ST Segment Depression

- Myocardial ischemia, left ventricular hypertrophy
- Intraventricular conduction defects
- Medication (e.g., digitalis)
- Reciprocal changes in leads opposite the area of acute injury

Notes:

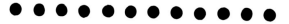

The Normal 12-Lead ECG

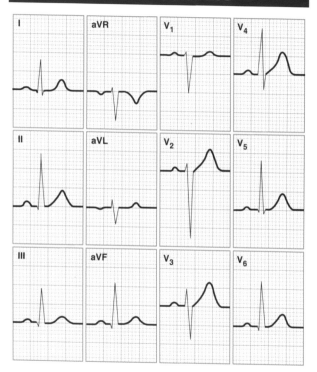

♥ **Clinical Tip:** A normal ECG does not rule out an acute coronary syndrome.

Anterior Myocardial Infarction

- Occlusion of the left coronary artery—left anterior descending branch
- ECG changes: ST segment elevation with tall T waves and taller-than-normal R waves in leads V_3 and V_4; reciprocal changes in II, III, and aVF

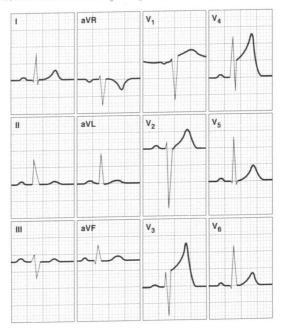

♥ **Clinical Tip:** Anterior MI frequently involves a large area of the myocardium and can present with cardiogenic shock, second-degree AV block type II, or third-degree AV block.

Inferior Myocardial Infarction

- Occlusion of the right coronary artery—posterior descending branch
- ECG changes: ST segment elevation in leads II, III, and aVF; reciprocal ST segment depression in I and aVL

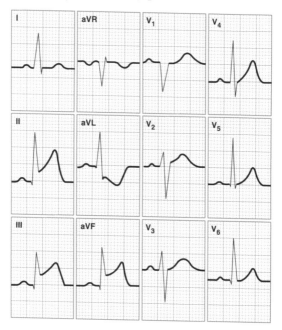

♥ **Clinical Tip:** Be alert for symptomatic sinus bradycardia, AV blocks, hypotension, and hypoperfusion.

Lateral Myocardial Infarction

- Occlusion of the left coronary artery—circumflex branch
- ECG changes: ST segment elevation in leads I, aVL, V_5, and V_6; reciprocal ST segment depression in V_1, V_2, and V_3

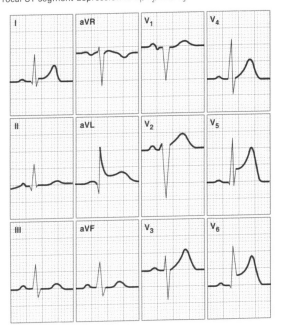

💜 **Clinical Tip:** Lateral MI is often associated with anterior or inferior wall MI. Be alert for changes that may indicate cardiogenic shock or congestive heart failure.

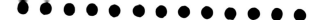

Septal Myocardial Infarction

- Occlusion of the left coronary artery—left anterior descending branch
- ECG changes: pathological Q waves; absence of normal R waves in leads V_1 and V_2

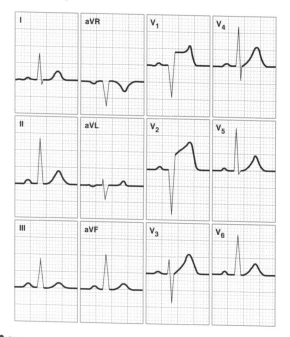

♥ **Clinical Tip:** Septal MI is often associated with an anterior wall MI.

Posterior Myocardial Infarction

- Occlusion of the right coronary artery (posterior descending branch) or the left circumflex artery
- Usually, tall R waves and ST segment depression in leads V_1, V_2, V_3, and V_4; possible left ventricular dysfunction
- You may need to view the true posterior leads, V_8 and V_9 (used in the 15-lead ECG), for definite diagnosis of an acute posterior MI. These leads show ST segment elevation.

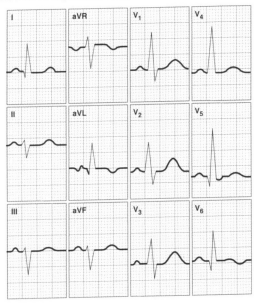

♥ **Clinical Tip:** Diagnosis may require a 15-lead ECG because a standard 12-lead does not look directly at the posterior wall.

Left Bundle Branch Block

- QRS complex greater than 0.10 sec
- QRS predominantly negative in leads V_1 and V_2
- QRS predominantly positive in V_5 and V_6 and often notched
- Absence of small, normal Q waves in I, aVL, V_5, and V_6
- Wide monophasic R waves in I, aVL, V_1, V_5, and V_6

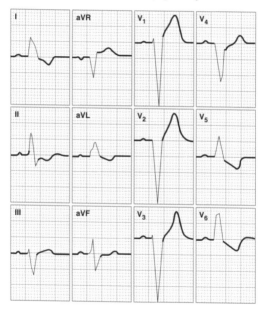

♥ **Clinical Tip:** Patients may have underlying heart disease, including coronary artery disease, hypertension, cardiomyopathy, and ischemia.

Right Bundle Branch Block

- QRS complex greater than 0.10 sec
- QRS axis normal or deviated to the right
- Broad S wave in leads I, aVL, V_5, and V_6
- RSR' pattern in lead V_1 with R' taller than R
- qRS pattern in V_5 and V_6
- ST segment to T wave distorted and in opposite direction to terminal portion of QRS (this is not ST elevation or ST depression)

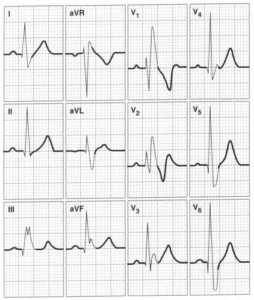

♥ **Clinical Tip**: Patients may have underlying right ventricular hypertrophy, pulmonary edema, cardiomyopathy, congenital heart disease, or rheumatic heart disease.

100

Emergency Medications

This is a reference list only. It is not meant to be exhaustive in clinical content. Drug dosages follow Advanced Cardiac Life Support (ACLS) guidelines for adult patients and Pediatric Advanced Life Support (PALS) guidelines for pediatric patients.

Before administering medications, especially IV medications, always consult an authoritative, current reference about dose, dilution, route, rate of administration, and interactions. Have a second licensed person independently check dose calculations, preparation, original orders, and infusion pump programming.

ACE Inhibitors

Class: Angiotensin-converting enzyme inhibitors.

Common Agents: Captopril, enalapril, lisinopril, ramipril.

Indications: MI, especially with ST elevation and with left ventricular dysfunction; HTN; heart failure without hypotension.

Adult Dose: See individual order and drug for route and dosage. Usually not started in the emergency department for an acute MI, but within 24 hr after reperfusion therapy has been completed and BP has stabilized.

Contraindications: Lactation, pregnancy, angioedema, hypersensitivity to ACE inhibitors, hypotension.

Side Effects: Cough, dizziness, headache, fatigue, hypotension, hyperkalemia, renal insufficiency.

Precautions: Reduce dose in renal failure. Caution in severe aortic stenosis, hypertrophic cardiomyopathy, unstented renal artery stenosis, severe CHF.

Adenosine (Adenocard)

Class: Antiarrhythmic.

Indications: Regular narrow-complex tachycardias, PSVT, and wide-complex tachycardia only if regular and monomorphic.

Adult Dose: 6 mg IV in the antecubital or another large vein given rapidly over 1–3 sec followed by a 20-mL bolus of normal saline. If the rhythm does not convert, give 12 mg by rapid IVP in 1–2 min if needed. A third dose of 12 mg IVP may be given in another 1–2 min, maximum (max) total dose 30 mg.

Adenosine (continued)

Pediatric Dose: 0.1 mg/kg (max 6 mg) IV/IO given rapidly over 1–3 sec followed by a 5- to 10-mL bolus of normal saline. If the rhythm does not convert, give 0.2 mg/kg (max 12 mg) IV/IO in 1–2 min if needed.

Contraindications: Hypersensitivity, sick sinus syndrome, second- or third-degree AV block (unless a functioning pacemaker is present), A-fib/A-flutter with underlying Wolff-Parkinson-White syndrome, drug- or poison-induced tachycardia, bronchospastic lung disease.

Side Effects: Flushing; nausea; dizziness; headache; dyspnea; bronchospasm; chest pain or tightness; discomfort in neck, throat, or jaw; bradycardia; AV block; asystole; ventricular ectopic beats; VF.

Precautions: Ineffective in treating A-fib, A-flutter, or VT. Less effective in patients taking theophylline or caffeine. Reduce dose in patients taking dipyridamole or carbamazepine or heart transplant patients.

Adenosine Diphosphate (ADP) Antagonists

Class: Antiplatelet agents—thienopyridines (clopidogrel and prasugrel), cyclopentyltriazolopyrimidine (ticagrelor).

Common Agents: Clopidogrel (Plavix), prasugrel (Effient), ticagrelor (Brilinta).

Indications: Antiplatelet therapy for acute coronary syndromes (ACS) managed with percutaneous coronary intervention (PCI). Clopidogrel: ACS, recent stroke, or peripheral arterial disease.

Adult Dose: See individual order and drug for dosage.

Contraindications: Acute pathological bleeding (e.g., peptic ulcer, intracranial bleeding). Prasugrel: Also history of TIA or stroke. Ticagrelor: Also history of intracranial hemorrhage, hepatic impairment.

Side Effects: Bleeding, thrombocytopenia purpura. Ticagrelor: Dyspnea, increased serum creatinine. Stent thrombosis with premature discontinuation of therapy.

Precautions: Increased risk of bleeding (chronic NSAID use, anticoagulation therapy, thrombocytopenia, trauma/surgery), thienopyridine hypersensitivity, severe hepatic impairment, severe renal impairment. Prasugrel: Caution in patients ≥75 years old or patients <60 kg. Ticagrelor: Patients with hyperuricemia or gouty arthritis, patients at risk for bradycardia without pacemaker. Drugs must be withheld prior to CABG or elective surgery—Clopidogrel and ticagrelor: 5 days; prasugrel: 7 days. In patients at risk for stent thrombosis, consider bridging with IV glycoprotein IIb/IIIa inhibitor such as eptifibatide (Integrilin)

while patient is off ADP antagonist; resume oral therapy as soon as possible after surgery when risk for postoperative bleeding is reduced.

Albuterol (ProAir, Proventil, Ventolin)

Class: Adrenergic beta$_2$-agonist, bronchodilator.

Indications: Asthma, COPD, anaphylaxis (bronchospasm), hyperkalemia.

Adult Dose: *For bronchospasm,* metered-dose inhaler (MDI): 2 puffs every 4–6 hr prn; nebulizer: 2.5 mg 3–4 times daily prn or 1.25–5 mg every 4–8 hr prn. *For severe bronchospasm and status asthmaticus:* 5 mcg/min IV, titrate up every 15–30 min to 10–20 mcg/min. For severe acute asthma exacerbation, MDI: 4–8 puffs every 20 min up to 4 hr, then every 1–4 hr prn; nebulizer: 2.5–5 mg every 20 min for 3 doses, then 2.5–10 mg every 1–4 hr prn or 10–15 mg/hr by continuous nebulizer.

Pediatric Dose: *For bronchospasm,* MDI 2 puffs every 4–6 hr prn; nebulizer children 2–12 yr: 0.63–1.25 mg 3–4 times daily prn; nebulizer children ≥12 yr: 2.5 mg 3–4 times daily prn. *For mild to moderate asthma or anaphylaxis, hyperkalemia,* MDI: 4–8 puffs every 20 min prn; nebulizer, <20 kg: 2.5 mg every 20 min, >20 kg: 5 mg every 20 min. *For severe asthma exacerbation,* MDI children <12 yr: 4–8 puffs every 20 min for 3 doses, then every 1–4 hr prn; MDI children ≥12 yr: 4–8 puffs every 20 min for up to 4 hr, then every 1–4 hr prn; nebulizer children <12 yr: 0.15 mg/kg every 20 min for 3 doses, then 0.15–0.3 mg/kg every 1–4 hr prn, or 0.5 mg/kg/hr by continuous nebulizer; nebulizer children ≥12 yr: 2.5–5 mg every 20 min for 3 doses, then 2.5–10 mg ever 1–4 hr prn, or 10–15 mg/hr by continuous nebulizer.

Contraindications: Hypersensitivity, tachyarrhythmias, risk of abortion during first or second trimester.

Side Effects: Angina, arrhythmias, palpitations, tachycardia, flushing, dizziness, headache, insomnia, irritability, angioedema, rash, urticaria, hypokalemia, hyperglycemia, asthma exacerbation, cough.

Precautions: Use of spacer with MDI is recommended. Caution in cardiovascular disease (arrhythmias, HTN, heart failure), diabetes (may increase serum glucose), glaucoma (increased intraocular pressure), hyperthyroidism (may stimulate thyroid activity), hypokalemia (decreased serum potassium), seizure disorders (CNS stimulation/excitation).

Amiodarone (Cordarone, Pacerone)

Class: Antiarrhythmic, class III.

Indications: Management of life-threatening shock-refractory VF or VT, recurrent hemodynamically unstable VT. Conversion of A-fib, SVT. Control of rapid ventricular rate in pre-excited atrial arrhythmias. Control of hemodynamically stable VT, polymorphic VT with normal QT interval, or wide-complex tachycardia of uncertain origin.

Adult Dose: *Cardiac arrest:* 300 mg IV/IO; consider additional 150 mg IV/IO in 3–5 min if needed. *Wide- and narrow-complex tachycardia (stable):* 150 mg IV over first 10 min (15 mg/min)—may repeat infusion of 150 mg IV every 10 min as needed; slow infusion of 360 mg IV over next 6 hr (1 mg/min); maintenance infusion of 540 mg over next 18 hr (0.5 mg/min). Max cumulative dose 2.2 g IV in 24 hr.

Pediatric Dose: *Cardiac arrest:* 5 mg/kg IV/IO bolus (max 300 mg), may repeat to max of 15 mg/kg (or 2.2 g in adolescents) in 24 hr; *Wide- and narrow-complex tachycardia (stable):* 5 mg/kg IV/IO load over 20–60 min (max 300 mg), may repeat to max of 15 mg/kg/day (2.2 g/day in adolescents).

Contraindications: Hypersensitivity, cardiogenic shock, symptomatic bradycardia or second- or third-degree AV block without functioning pacemaker, severe sinus node dysfunction.

Side Effects: Vasodilation, hypotension, bradycardia, proarrhythmic effects, visual impairment, hepatotoxicity, pulmonary toxicity, CHF. May prolong QT interval, producing torsade de pointes.

Precautions: Avoid concurrent use with procainamide. Correct hypokalemia and hypomagnesemia, if possible, before use. Draw up amiodarone through a large-gauge needle to reduce foaming. For slow or maintenance IV infusion, mix the medication only in a glass bottle containing D5W or NS and administer through an in-line filter using a volumetric pump. Use with caution in thyroid disease, pulmonary disease, or hepatic impairment, and in patients on warfarin.

Aspirin (Acetylsalicylic Acid, ASA)

Class: Antiplatelet.

Indications: Acute coronary syndrome, symptoms suggestive of cardiac ischemia, post-percutaneous coronary interventions, A-fib, stroke, peripheral arterial disease.

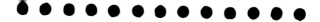

Adult Dose: *Acute coronary syndrome*: 160–325 mg PO. Chewing the tablet is preferable; use non–enteric-coated tablets for more rapid antiplatelet effect. Give within minutes of onset of ischemic symptoms. Other indications: 81–325 mg PO daily.

Contraindications: Known allergy to aspirin, third trimester of pregnancy, bleeding.

Side Effects: Anorexia, nausea, epigastric pain, bleeding, anaphylaxis.

Precautions: GERD, active ulcers, asthma, bleeding disorders, or thrombocytopenia.

Atropine Sulfate

Class: Anticholinergic, parasympatholytic, vagolytic.

Indications: Symptomatic sinus bradycardia, junctional escape rhythm, or second-degree type I block. Not likely to be effective in second-degree type II or third-degree AV block with wide QRS complex.

Adult Dose: 0.5 mg IV given every 3–5 min as needed, max total dose 3 mg (0.04 mg/kg).

Pediatric Dose: 0.02 mg/kg IV/IO (min. dose 0.1 mg, max single dose child 0.5 mg, max single dose adolescent 1 mg), may repeat dose once, max total dose child 1 mg, max total dose adolescent 3 mg. May give 0.04–0.06 mg/kg, flush with 5 mL normal saline if administering by ET. Use ET route only if IV/IO access is not available.

Contraindications: Hypersensitivity, acute angle-closure glaucoma, asthma, prostatic hypertrophy, myasthenia gravis.

Side Effects: Tachycardia, headache, dry mouth, nausea, constipation, dilated pupils, flushing, hypotension.

Precautions: Use caution in myocardial ischemia and hypoxia. Avoid in hypothermic bradycardia and in second-degree (Mobitz type II) and third-degree AV block with wide QRS complex, asystole, bradycardic PEA. Caution in colon disease, hepatic or renal impairment, hiatal hernia, obstructive uropathy, hyperthyroidism.

Beta Blockers

Class: Beta blockers, antihypertensive, antiarrhythmic, antianginal.

Common Agents: Atenolol, esmolol, labetalol, metoprolol, propranolol.

Indications: MI, unstable angina, PSVT, A-fib, A-flutter, HTN, CHF.

Adult Dose: See individual order and drug for route and dosage.

Beta Blockers (continued)

Contraindications: Heart rate <50 bpm, systolic BP <100 mm Hg, second- or third-degree AV block or sick sinus syndrome without functioning pacemaker, severe decompensated left ventricular failure, cardiogenic shock. Nonselective beta blockers are contraindicated in bronchospastic disease.

Side Effects: Hypotension, dizziness, bradycardia, headache, fatigue, nausea and vomiting, depression.

Precautions: Concurrent use with calcium channel blockers, such as verapamil or diltiazem, can cause hypotension. Use beta-1 selective agents with caution in patients with a history of bronchospasm. Use caution in thyroid disease, peripheral arterial disease, and diabetes (monitor blood glucose levels frequently).

Calcium Chloride

Class: Minerals, electrolytes, calcium salt.

Indications: Hyperkalemia, hypocalcemia, hypermagnesemia; antidote for calcium channel blocker or beta blocker overdose.

Adult Dose: 500–1000 mg (5–10 mL of a 10% solution) over 2–5 min IV; may be repeated as needed.

Pediatric Dose: 20 mg/kg (0.2 mL/kg) IV/IO slow push during arrest or if severe hypotension, repeat as needed.

Contraindications: Hypercalcemia, hypophosphatemia, VF, digoxin toxicity.

Side effects: Bradycardia, hypotension, hypomagnesemia, hypercalcemia, VF, syncope, nephrolithiasis, flushing, dizziness, nausea and vomiting.

Precautions: Incompatible with sodium bicarbonate (precipitates). Caution in patients with renal impairment, respiratory acidosis, hypokalemia, hyperparathyroidism.

Digoxin (Lanoxin)

Class: Antiarrhythmic, cardiac glycoside.

Indications: To slow ventricular response in A-fib or A-flutter; rarely, as a positive inotrope in CHF.

Adult Dose: Loading dose of 0.5 mg IV over 5 min, 0.25 mg IV in 6–8 hr × 2. Maintenance dose determined by body size and renal function.

Contraindications: Hypersensitivity, uncontrolled ventricular arrhythmias, AV block without functioning pacemaker, idiopathic hypertrophic subaortic stenosis (IHSS), constrictive pericarditis, A-fib with Wolff-Parkinson-White syndrome.

Side Effects: Accelerated junctional rhythm, atrial tachycardia with block, AV block, asystole, VT, VF, ventricular bigeminy and trigeminy, dizziness, weakness, fatigue, nausea and vomiting, blurred or yellow vision, headache, hypersensitivity, hypokalemia.

Precautions: Avoid electrical cardioversion of stable patients. If the patient's condition is unstable, use lower current settings such as 10–20 J. Use cautiously in elderly patients and patients with heart failure, acute MI, renal impairment, and hypothyroidism. Correct electrolyte abnormalities, monitor digoxin levels, monitor for clinical signs of toxicity. Hypokalemia, hypomagnesemia, and hypercalcemia may precipitate digitalis toxicity. Reduce digoxin dose by 50% in patients on amiodarone.

Digoxin Immune FAB (Fragment Antigen Binding) (DigiFab)

Class: Antidote to digoxin and digitoxin.

Indications: Symptomatic digoxin toxicity or acute ingestion of unknown amount of digoxin.

Adult Dose: Depends on serum digoxin levels. One 40-mg vial binds to approximately 0.5 mg of digoxin. Dose is typically administered over 30 min.

Contraindications: Allergy only, otherwise none known. Allergy to sheep proteins or other sheep products.

Side Effects: Worsening of CHF, rapid ventricular response in patients with A-fib, hypokalemia, postural hypotension, increased serum digoxin levels due to bound complexes (clinically misleading because bound complex cannot interact with receptors).

Precautions: Heart failure, renal impairment.

Diltiazem (Cardizem)

Class: Calcium channel blocker, antiarrhythmic, class IV.

Indications: To control ventricular rate in A-fib and A-flutter; to terminate PSVT (reentry SVT) refractory to adenosine with narrow QRS complex and adequate BP.

Adult Dose: 15–20 mg (0.25 mg/kg) IV given over 2 min. May repeat in 15 min at 20–25 mg (0.35 mg/kg) IV given over 2 min. Start maintenance drip at 5–15 mg/hr and titrate to HR.

Contraindications: Drug- or poison-induced tachycardia, wide-complex tachycardia of uncertain origin, rapid A-fib and A-flutter with Wolff-Parkinson-White syndrome, sick sinus syndrome, second- or third-degree

Diltiazem (continued)

AV block (unless a functioning pacemaker is present), hypotension with systolic BP less than 90 mm Hg, acute MI with pulmonary congestion.

Side Effects: Hypotension, bradycardia (including AV block), chest pain, ventricular arrhythmias, peripheral edema, flushing, heart failure, syncope.

Precautions: Severe hypotension in patients receiving beta blockers. Caution in patients with hepatic or renal disease, heart failure, hypertrophic cardiomyopathy.

Dobutamine

Class: Adrenergic direct-acting beta$_1$-agonist, inotrope.

Indications: To increase myocardial contractility in patients with decompensated heart failure with systolic BP 70–100 mm Hg and no signs of shock.

Adult Dose: Continuous infusion (titrate to patient response): 2–20 mcg/kg/min, max 40 mcg/kg/min.

Pediatric Dose: Same as adult dose, titrate to patient response.

Contraindications: Hypersensitivity, idiopathic hypertrophic subaortic stenosis (IHSS), suspected or known poison- or drug-induced shock. Do not mix with sodium bicarbonate.

Side Effects: Tachycardia, HTN, hypotension, increased ventricular ectopy, chest pain, palpitations, restlessness, headache, nausea, vomiting.

Precautions: Avoid in patients with systolic BP <100 mm Hg and signs of shock; correct hypovolemia before use, if needed. MI: may increase myocardial oxygen demand.

Dopamine (Intropin)

Class: Alpha-and beta$_1$-adrenergic agonist, inotrope, vasopressor.

Indications: Symptomatic bradycardia and hypotension, cardiogenic shock.

Adult Dose: Continuous infusion (titrate to patient response): low dose 1–5 mcg/kg/min (renal dose); moderate dose 5–10 mcg/kg/min (cardiac dose); high dose 10–20 mcg/kg/min (vasopressor dose). Mix 400 mg/250 mL in normal saline, lactated Ringer's solution, or D5W (1600 mcg/mL).

Pediatric Dose: *Cardiogenic shock, distributive shock:* 2–20 mcg/kg/min IV/IO infusion, titrate to desired effect.

Contraindications: Hypersensitivity to sulfites, pheochromocytoma, VF.

Side Effects: Tachyarrhythmias, angina, hypotension, palpitations, vasoconstriction, dyspnea, headache, nausea and vomiting.

Precautions: Hypovolemia, MI. Adjust dosage in elderly patients and in those with occlusive vascular disease. Ensure adequate IV volume repletion with normal saline before infusion. Taper slowly. Do not mix with sodium bicarbonate. Use care with peripheral administration; infiltration with extravasation can cause tissue necrosis. A central line is preferred. Use a volumetric infusion pump. Caution in patients with occlusive vascular disease and patients taking MAO inhibitors.

Epinephrine (Adrenalin)

Class: Alpha-beta adrenergic agonist (sympathomimetic: inotrope, vasopressor, bronchodilator).

Indications: Cardiac arrest: PEA, asystole, pulseless VT, VF; hypotension with severe bradycardia. Anaphylaxis, severe asthma exacerbation.

Adult Dose: *Cardiac arrest:* 1 mg IV/IO (10 mL of 1:10,000 solution) every 3–5 min prn; follow each dose with 20 mL IV flush. Give 2.0–2.5 mg diluted in 10 mL normal saline or sterile water if administering by ET tube. *Profound bradycardia or hypotension:* 2–10 mcg/min IV infusion; add 1 mg (1 mL of a 1:1000 solution) to 500 mL normal saline or D5W. *Anaphylaxis:* 0.2–0.5 mg (1:1000 solution) IM (1:1000 solution) every 5–15 min prn or 0.1–0.25 mg (1:10,000 solution) IV every 5–15 min, then 1–4 mcg/min IV prn. *Severe asthma exacerbation:* 0.3–0.5 mg (1:1000 solution) SQ/IM every 20 min × 3 doses prn. Max 1 mg/dose.

Pediatric Dose: *Cardiac arrest or symptomatic bradycardia:* 0.01 mg/kg (0.1 mL/kg) 1:10,000 IV/IO every 3–5 min as needed (max 1 mg; 10 mL). Give 0.1 mg/kg (0.1 mL/kg) 1:1000, flush with 5 mL normal saline if administering by ET tube. Use ET route only if IV/IO access is not available. Repeat every 3–5 min as needed. *Anaphylaxis:* 0.01 mg/kg (1:1000 solution) SQ/IM every 5–20 min × 3 doses prn or 0.01 mg/kg (1:10,000 solution) IV × 1, then 0.1 mcg/kg/min IV prn. *Severe asthma exacerbation:* 0.01 mg/kg (1:1000 solution) SQ/IM every 20 min × 3 doses prn. Max 0.5 mg/dose.

Contraindications: Hypersensitivity to adrenergic amines, hypovolemic shock, coronary insufficiency. No contraindication in cardiac arrest.

Side Effects: Angina, HTN, tachycardia, VT, VF, nervousness, restlessness, palpitations, tremors, weakness, diaphoresis, anxiety, headache, nausea.

Epinephrine (continued)

Precautions: Use caution in HTN and increasing heart rate (may cause increased myocardial oxygen demand). Higher doses can contribute to post-arrest cardiac impairment but may be needed to treat poison- or drug-induced shock. Avoid mixing with alkaline solutions.

Fibrinolytic Agents

Class: Thrombolytic, fibrinolytic.

Common Agents: Alteplase (Activase, t-PA), reteplase (Retavase), streptokinase (Streptase), tenecteplase (TNKase).

Indications: Acute ST elevation MI within the past 12 hr. Alteplase is the only fibrinolytic agent approved for acute ischemic stroke and must be started less than 3 hr from the onset of symptoms.

Adult Dose: See individual order and drug for route and dosage.

Contraindications: Active internal bleeding within 21 days (except menses), neurovascular event within 3 months, major surgery or trauma within 2 weeks, aortic dissection, severe (uncontrolled) HTN, bleeding disorders, prolonged CPR, lumbar puncture within 1 week. History of any intracranial bleeding, oral anticoagulation therapy, severe stroke.

Side Effects: Hypotension, reperfusion arrhythmias, heart failure, headache, increased bleeding time, deep or superficial hemorrhage, flushing, urticaria, anaphylaxis.

Precautions: Use cautiously in patients with severe renal or hepatic disease. Initiate bleeding precautions. Monitor patient for bleeding complications.

Fondaparinux (Arixtra)

Class: Factor Xa inhibitor, anticoagulant.

Indications: To inhibit thrombin generation by inhibiting factor Xa in patients with ACS; anticoagulation in patients with history of heparin-induced thrombocytopenia (HIT); deep vein thrombosis (DVT) prophylaxis in patients undergoing orthopedic surgery or abdominal surgery; pulmonary embolism (PE); acute DVT without PE.

Adult Dose: *STEMI:* 2.5 mg IV bolus followed by 2.5 mg SQ daily for up to 8 days. *Acute DVT/PE, acute thrombosis:* 5–10 mg SQ daily (based on body weight) up to 5–9 days, start coumadin therapy on first or second day, discontinue fondaparinux when INR ≥2 for at least 24 hr. *Other uses:* 2.5 mg SQ daily for up to 8 days (up to 10 days for abdominal surgery, up to 11 days for hip replacement or total knee replacement surgery, up to 14 days for total hip or total knee arthroplasty or hip fracture surgery).

Contraindications: Creatinine clearance <30 mL/min, hypersensitivity, body weight <50 kg when used for prophylaxis, active major bleeding, bacterial endocarditis, thrombocytopenia associated with positive *in vitro* test for antiplatelet antibody in presence of fondaparinux.

Side Effects: Bleeding, edema, hypotension, insomnia, dizziness, headache, rash, constipation, vomiting, diarrhea, urinary retention, moderate thrombocytopenia.

Precautions: Increased risk of bleeding, creatinine clearance 30–50 mL/min, patients >75 years old, patients <50 kg being treated for DVT/PE. Discontinue 24 hr before CABG and administer unfractionated heparin.

Furosemide (Lasix)

Class: Loop diuretic.

Indications: CHF with acute pulmonary edema, hypertensive crisis, post-arrest cerebral edema, edema associated with hepatic or renal disease.

Adult Dose: 0.5–1 mg/kg IV given over 1–2 min; may repeat at 2 mg/kg IV given over 1–2 min. Alternative: 20–40 mg IV, increase by 20 mg IV every 2 hr until desired response is obtained, max 160–200 mg/dose.

Pediatric Dose: 0.5–1 mg/kg IV/IO, may increase by 1 mg/kg IV every 2 hr until desired response is obtained, max 6 mg/kg/dose.

Contraindications: Hypersensitivity (cross-sensitivity with thiazides and sulfonamides may occur), uncontrolled electrolyte imbalance, hepatic coma, anuria, hypovolemia.

Side Effects: Severe dehydration, hypovolemia, hypotension, hypokalemia, hyponatremia, hypochloremia, hyperglycemia, dizziness, ototoxicity.

Precautions: Use cautiously in severe liver disease accompanied by cirrhosis or ascites, electrolyte depletion, diabetes mellitus, pregnancy, lactation, severe renal disease, gout. Risk for ototoxicity with increased dose or rapid injection. Monitor electrolytes closely.

Glycoprotein IIB/IIIA Inhibitors

Class: Antiplatelet agents, GP IIb/IIIa inhibitors.

Common Agents: Abciximab (ReoPro), eptifibatide (Integrilin), tirofiban (Aggrastat).

Glycoprotein IIB/IIIA Inhibitors (continued)

Indications: Acute coronary syndromes managed medically (Eptifibatide and Tirofiban) and those undergoing PCI (all three agents).

Adult Dose: See individual order and drug for dosage.

Contraindications: Hypersensitivity, active internal bleeding or bleeding disorder within past 30 days, history of bleeding diathesis, history of stroke within 30 days, history of hemorrhagic stroke, uncontrolled HTN (systolic BP >200 mm Hg, diastolic pressure >110 mm Hg), major surgery or trauma within 1 month, concomitant use of another GP IIb/IIIa inhibitor, dependency on hemodialysis.

Side Effects: Bleeding, hypotension, thrombocytopenia.

Precautions: Patients at increased risk for bleeding, patients <70 kg, platelet count <150,000/mm³, renal impairment. Discontinue ≥2–4 hr prior to CABG. Abciximab (ReoPro) must be administered with aspirin and heparin.

Heparin (Unfractionated Heparin [UFH])

Class: Anticoagulant.

Indications: Acute coronary syndromes (ACS): STEMI, NSTEMI, unstable angina (UA), during PCI; prophylaxis and treatment of thromboembolic disorders such as DVT, pulmonary embolus; anticoagulant for extracorporeal and dialysis procedures.

Adult Dose: *ACS:* 60 units/kg IV bolus, max 4000 units, followed by continuous IV infusion of 12 units/kg/hr, max 1000 units/hr, check APTT every 4–6 hr, adjust infusion to maintain APTT 50–70 sec for 48 hr or until angiography. *Thromboprophylaxis:* 5000 units SQ every 8–12 hr. Treatment of DVT/PE: 80 units/kg or 5000 unit IV bolus, followed by continuous IV infusion of 18 units/kg/hr; adjust infusion to maintain therapeutic APTT.

Pediatric Dose: *Systemic heparinization for infants <1 year:* 75 units/kg IV over 10 min, followed by initial maintenance infusion of 28 units/kg/hr; check APTT every 4 hr and adjust heparin dose to maintain APTT 60–85 sec. *For children >1 year:* 75 units/kg over 10 min, followed by initial maintenance infusion of 20 units/kg/hr, adjust heparin to maintain APTT 60–85 sec.

Contraindications: Hypersensitivity, heparin-induced thrombocytopenia (HIT), severe thrombocytopenia, uncontrolled active bleeding unless due to DIC; recent intracranial, intraspinal, or eye surgery; uncontrolled HTN.

Side Effects: Bleeding, HIT, thrombocytopenia, hyperkalemia, osteoporosis with use >6 mo.

Precautions: Patients at increased risk for bleeding; patients with heparin resistance (antithrombin deficiency, increased heparin clearance elevations in heparin-binding proteins, elevations in factor VIII and/or fibrinogen). Female patients >60 yr old may require lower doses. Check platelet count daily.

Ibutilide (Corvert)

Class: Antiarrhythmic, class III.

Indications: SVT, including A-fib and A-flutter; most effective for conversion of A-fib or A-flutter of short duration (≤48 hr).

Adult Dose: *Patients weighing 60 kg or more:* 1 mg IV given over 10 min; may repeat the same dose in 10 min if arrhythmia does not terminate. *Patients weighing <60 kg:* 0.01 mg/kg IV given over 10 min; may repeat the same dose in 10 min if arrhythmia does not terminate.

Contraindications: Known hypersensitivity, history of polymorphic VT, QTc greater than 440 msec.

Side Effects: Nonsustained or sustained monomorphic or polymorphic VT, torsade de pointes, AV block, CHF, HTN, headache, tachycardia, hypotension, nausea and vomiting.

Precautions: Continuous ECG monitoring for 4–6 hr after administration or until QTc returns to baseline. Monitor for AV block. Skilled personnel and resuscitative equipment must be readily available. Correct electrolyte abnormalities prior to use. If A-fib has lasted longer than 48 hr, anticoagulation is required before cardioversion with ibutilide. Monitor QTc. Not recommended for chronic atrial fibrillation. Caution in patients with heart failure or hepatic impairment.

Isoproterenol (Isuprel)

Class: Beta-adrenergic agonist.

Indications: Medically refractory symptomatic bradycardia when transcutaneous or transvenous pacing is not available, refractory torsade de pointes unresponsive to magnesium, bradycardia in heart transplant patients, beta blocker poisoning.

Adult Dose: IV infusion: mix 1 mg/250 mL in normal saline, lactated Ringer's solution, or D5W, run at 2–10 mcg/min, and titrate to patient response. In torsade de pointes, titrate to increase heart rate until VT is suppressed.

Isoproterenol (continued)

Contraindications: Hypersensitivity to drug or sulfites, digitalis intoxication, angina, tachyarrhythmias, concurrent use with epinephrine (can cause VF or VT).

Side Effects: Arrhythmias, cardiac arrest, hypotension, angina, anxiety, tachycardia, palpitations, skin flushing, dizziness, tremors, headache, nausea, vomiting, restlessness.

Precautions: May increase myocardial ischemia. Use caution in patients with renal impairment, cardiovascular disease, distributive shock, hyperthyroidism, diabetes. High doses are harmful except in beta blocker overdose.

Lidocaine (Xylocaine)

Class: Antiarrhythmic, class Ib, local anesthetic.

Indications: Alternative to amiodarone in VF or pulseless VT. Use in stable VT, wide-complex tachycardia of uncertain origin.

Adult Dose: *Cardiac arrest from VF or VT:* 1.0–1.5 mg/kg IV/IO (or 2–4 mg/kg via ET tube); may repeat 0.5–0.75 mg/kg IV/IO every 5–10 min, max dose 3 mg/kg. *Stable VT, wide-complex tachycardia of uncertain origin:* 0.50–0.75 mg/kg up to 1.0–1.5 mg/kg; may repeat 0.50–0.75 mg/kg every 5–10 min, max total dose 3.0 mg/kg. If conversion is successful, start an IV infusion of 1–4 mg/min (30–50 mcg/kg/min) in normal saline or D5W.

Pediatric Dose: 1 mg/kg IV/IO bolus. Give 2–3 mg/kg, flush with 5 mL normal saline if administering by ET tube. Use ET route only if IV/IO access is not available. Maintenance: 20–50 mcg/kg/min IV/IO infusion (repeat bolus [0.5–1 mg/kg IV/IO] when infusion is initiated if bolus has not been given within previous 15 min).

Contraindications: Prophylactic use in acute MI, advanced AV block without functioning pacemaker, hypotension, Wolff-Parkinson-White syndrome, hypersensitivity to amide local anesthetics.

Side Effects: Confusion, agitation, anxiety, tinnitus, blurred vision, dizziness, tremors, hallucinations, seizures, hypotension, bradycardia, cardiovascular collapse, respiratory arrest, slurred speech.

Precautions: CHF, respiratory depression, shock. Reduce maintenance dose (not loading dose) in presence of impaired liver function or left ventricular dysfunction or in the elderly. Stop infusion if signs of CNS toxicity develop.

Magnesium Sulfate

Class: Electrolyte, antiarrhythmic.

Indications: Torsade de pointes, hypomagnesemia, life-threatening ventricular arrhythmias due to digitalis toxicity, status asthmaticus, seizures.

Adult Dose: *Torsade de pointes (cardiac arrest):* 1–2 g IV (2–4 mL of a 50% solution) diluted in 10 mL of D5W over 1–2 min. *Torsade de pointes (non–cardiac arrest with pulse):* load with 1–2 g mixed in 50–100 mL of D5W infused over 5–60 min IV, then infuse 0.5–1.0 g/hr IV (titrate to control torsade). *Seizures:* 2 g IV diluted in 10 mL of D5W over 10 min.

Pediatric Dose: *Torsade de pointes (cardiac arrest—pulseless VT):* 25–50 mg/kg IV/IO bolus. *Torsade de pointes (non–cardiac arrest with pulses):* 25–50 mg/kg IV/IO over 10–20 min. *Status asthmaticus:* 25–50 mg/kg/IV/IO over 15–30 min.

Contraindications: Hypermagnesemia, hypocalcemia, AV block.

Side Effects: HTN, bradycardia, cardiac arrest, respiratory depression, altered LOC, flushed skin, diaphoresis, hypocalcemia, hyperkalemia, hypophosphatemia.

Precautions: Renal insufficiency, occasional fall in BP with rapid administration. Monitor serum magnesium levels. Caution in patients with myasthenia gravis. Correct concurrent hypokalemia and hypocalcemia.

Morphine Sulfate

Class: Opiate narcotic analgesic.

Indications: Chest pain unrelieved by nitroglycerin; CHF and dyspnea associated with pulmonary edema.

Adult Dose: 2–4 mg IV (given over 1–5 min), administer every 5–30 min as needed if hemodynamically stable; may repeat dose of 2–8 mg at 5- to 15-min intervals if needed.

Contraindications: Hypersensitivity, heart failure due to chronic lung disease, respiratory depression, hypercarbia, hypotension, bowel obstruction, severe asthma, acute or severe hypercarbia. Avoid in patients with RV infarction.

Side Effects: Respiratory depression, hypotension, nausea and vomiting, bradycardia, altered LOC, seizures, somnolence, dizziness, diaphoresis, flushing, pruritus, dry mouth, urinary retention.

Precautions: Administer slowly and titrate to effect. Reverse with naloxone (0.4–2.0 mg IV) if necessary. Use caution in cerebral edema

Morphine Sulfate (continued)

and pulmonary edema with compromised respiration. Use caution with hypovolemic patients; be prepared to administer volume. Use caution in renal and hepatic impairment, seizure disorder, CNS depression, head injury, hypothyroidism, adrenal insufficiency, prostatic hypertrophy, shock.

Naloxone (Narcan)

Class: Opioid antagonist.

Indications: Reversal of opioid overdose/toxicity unresponsive to oxygen and ventilator support, such as respiratory and neurological depression.

Adult dose: *Opioid overdose*: 2 mg IV, IM, or SQ; may need to repeat every 2-3 min up to 10 mg. Reversal of respiratory depression with therapeutic opioid doses: 0.04–0.4 mg IV, IM, or SQ; may repeat until ventilation is adequate, up to 0.8 mg. *Postoperative reversal*: 0.1–0.2 mg IV every 2–3 min until adequate ventilation.

Pediatric dose: *For total reversal, birth to 5 yr*: 0.1 mg/kg IV every 2–3 min as needed, max 2 mg; *>5 yr*: 2 mg IV every 2–3 min prn up to 10 mg. *For partial reversal*: 0.001–0.005 mg/kg IV (1–5 mcg/kg), repeat as needed every 2–3 min. *For postoperative reversal*: 0.01 mg/kg IV every 2–3 min prn.

Contraindications: Hypersensitivity, meperidine-induced seizures.

Side Effects: Secondary to reversal (withdrawal) of narcotic analgesia and sedation. Recurrent respiratory depression, pain, hypertension, hypotension, irritability, agitation, diaphoresis, seizures.

Precautions: May precipitate symptoms of acute withdrawal in opioid-dependent patients. Use caution in patients with a history of seizures and patients with cardiovascular disease. Abrupt postoperative reversal may cause nausea, vomiting, diaphoresis, tachycardia, hypertension, seizures, pulmonary edema, arrhythmias.

Nitroglycerin (Nitrostat, Nitrolingual [Pump spray])

Class: Antianginal, nitrate, vasodilator.

Indications: Acute coronary syndrome, angina, CHF associated with acute MI, hypertensive urgency with ACS.

Adult Dose: Sublingual route, 0.3–0.4 mg (1 tablet); repeat every 3–5 min if chest pain is not relieved, max 3 doses/15 min. Aerosol, spray for 0.5–1.0 sec at 3- to 5-min intervals (provides 0.4 mg/dose), max 3 sprays/15 min. IV bolus administration at 12.5–25.0 mcg (if no sublingual or

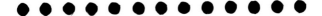

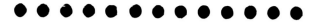

spray used). IV infusion: mix 25 mg/250 mL (100 mcg/mL) in D5W, start at 5 mcg/min and titrate by 5 mcg/min every 3–5 min to 20 mcg/min. If patient remains symptomatic, titrate by 10–20 mcg/min every 3–5 min, max 200 mcg/min.

Pediatric Dose: 0.25–0.50 mcg/kg/min IV/IO infusion, titrate by 0.5–1 mcg/kg/min every 3–5 min as needed to typical dose range of 1–5 mcg/kg/min (max 20 mcg/kg/min).

Contraindications: Hypersensitivity, systolic BP less than 90 mm Hg, pericardial tamponade, constrictive pericarditis, severe bradycardia or severe tachycardia associated with hypotension; sildenafil (Viagra) or vardenafil (Levitra) within 24 hr, tadalafil (Cialis) within 48 hr; right ventricular infarction, increased intracranial pressure, hypertrophic cardiomyopathy with outflow tract obstruction, restrictive cardiomyopathy, increased intracranial pressure.

Side Effects: Hypotension with reflex tachycardia, syncope, headache, flushed skin, dizziness, paradoxical bradycardia.

Precautions: Do not mix with other medications; titrate IV to maintain systolic BP above 90 mm Hg. Mix only in glass IV bottles and infuse only through non-PVC tubing; standard polyvinyl chloride (PVC) tubing can bind up to 80% of the medication, making it necessary to infuse higher doses. Do not shake aerosol spray (affects metered dose).

Norepinephrine (Levophed)

Class: Alpha- and beta-adrenergic agonist, vasopressor.

Indications: Treatment of persistent shock after adequate volume replacement, cardiogenic shock, low systemic vascular resistance shock, septic shock, hemodynamically significant hypotension.

Adult Dose: Start at 0.1–0.5 mcg/kg/min, titrate to response up to 8–12 mcg/min, maintenance infusion usually 2–4 mcg/min. Use volumetric infusion pump.

Pediatric Dose: Start at 0.05–0.1 mcg/kg/min, titrate to response, up to 2 mcg/kg/min. Use volumetric infusion pump.

Contraindications: Hypovolemic shock prior to adequate volume replacement, mesenteric or peripheral vascular thrombosis except as emergency measure to maintain coronary and cerebral perfusion. Do not administer in same line as alkaline solutions.

Side Effects: Arrhythmias, hypertension, headache, anxiety, dyspnea, skin necrosis with extravasation.

Norepinephrine (continued)

Precautions: Use caution in patients on MAO inhibitors as drug may cause prolonged hypertension; infuse into large vein and avoid extravasation; use caution in patients with ischemic heart disease: increases myocardial oxygen consumption, may induce arrhythmias, tachycardia, hypertension.

Oxygen

Class: Gas.

Indications: Cardiopulmonary emergencies with shortness of breath and chest pain, cardiac or respiratory arrest, hypoxemia. Used to optimize oxygen saturation <94%.

Adult and Pediatric Dose: Nasal cannula 1–6 L/min (21%–44% oxygen), Venturi mask 4–12 L/min (24%–50% oxygen), simple mask 5–8 L/min (40%–60% oxygen), partial rebreathing mask 6–10 L/min (35%–60% oxygen), non-rebreathing mask 6–15 L/min (60%–100% oxygen), bag-valve mask 15 L/min (95%–100% oxygen).

Contraindications: None reported.

Side Effects: Drying of respiratory mucosa, possible bronchospasm if oxygen is extremely cold and dry. Oxygen supports combustion and can fuel a fire. Hypoventilation in patients with severe COPD, pulmonary fibrosis, oxygen toxicity.

Precautions: Respiratory arrest in patients with hypoxic respiratory drive. The patient needs an airway and adequate ventilation before oxygen is effective.

Procainamide (Pronestyl)

Class: Antiarrhythmic, class I_a.

Indications: Recurrent VT or VF, PSVT refractory to adenosine and vagal stimulation, rapid A-fib with Wolff-Parkinson-White syndrome, stable wide-complex tachycardia of uncertain origin, maintenance after conversion. Stable monomorphic VT with normal QTc and preserved LV function.

Adult Dose: 20 mg/min IV infusion or up to 50 mg/min under urgent conditions, until arrhythmia is suppressed, max 17 mg/kg loading dose. Maintenance IV infusion: mix 1 g/250 mL (4 mg/mL) in normal saline or D5W, run at 1–4 mg/min.

Pediatric Dose: *Atrial flutter, SVT, VT (with pulses)*: 15 mg/kg IV/IO load over 30–60 min.

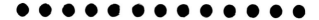

Contraindications: Hypersensitivity, second- and third-degree AV block (unless a functioning pacemaker is in place), prolonged QT interval, torsade de pointes, hypersensitivity, systemic lupus erythematosus.

Side Effects: Hypotension, widening QRS, headache, nausea and vomiting, flushed skin, seizures, ventricular arrhythmias, AV block, cardiovascular collapse, arrest.

Precautions: Monitor BP every 2–3 min while administering procainamide. If QRS width increases by 50% or more, or if systolic BP decreases to less than 90 mm Hg, stop the drug. Monitor for prolonged PR interval and AV block. Monitor for QT prolongation. May precipitate or exacerbate CHF. Reduce the total dose to 12 mg/kg and maintenance infusion to 1–2 mg/min if cardiac or renal dysfunction is present. Use cautiously in heart failure, myasthenia gravis, and hepatic or renal disease. Avoid concurrent use with drugs that prolong the QT interval (e.g., amiodarone, sotalol).

Sodium Bicarbonate

Class: Alkalinizing agent, buffer.

Indications: Known preexisting hyperkalemia, bicarbonate-responsive acidosis such as diabetic ketoacidosis or tricyclic antidepressant overdose, metabolic acidosis associated with prolonged resuscitation with effective ventilation.

Adult Dose: 1 mEq/kg IV; may repeat 0.5 mEq/kg every 10 min. Dosing is best guided by calculated base deficits or bicarbonate concentration with arterial blood gas analysis if available.

Pediatric Dose: 1 mEq/kg IV/IO slow bolus. Dosing is best guided by calculated base deficits or bicarbonate concentration with arterial blood gas analysis, if available.

Contraindications: Metabolic and respiratory alkalosis, hypochloremia, hypocalcemia, hypokalemia, hypercarbic acidosis, hypernatremia, severe pulmonary edema.

Side Effects: Hypokalemia, hypocalcemia, hypernatremia, metabolic alkalosis, edema, seizures, tetany, exacerbation of CHF, tissue hypoxia, intracellular acidosis.

Precautions: CHF, renal disease, cirrhosis, hypernatremia, hypervolemia, toxemia, concurrent corticosteroid therapy. Not recommended for routine use in cardiac arrest because adequate ventilation and CPR are the major "buffer agents" in this case. Incompatible with many drugs; flush the line before and after administration.

Vasopressin (Pitressin)

Class: Vasopressor, hormone.

Indication: Cardiac arrest: an alternative to epinephrine in shock-refractory VF and pulseless VT, PEA, and asystole. Vasodilatory shock/septic shock.

Adult Dose: *Cardiac arrest:* 40 units IV/IO single dose to replace first or second dose of epinephrine as an alternative. *Vasodilatory shock:* 0.01–0.04 units/min continuous IV infusion.

Pediatric Dose: *Cardiac arrest:* 0.4–1 unit/kg IV/IO, max 40 units. *Vasodilatory shock:* 0.0002–0.002 unit/kg/min continuous IV infusion.

Contraindications: Hypersensitivity.

Side Effects: Bradycardia, HTN, angina, MI, arrhythmias, dizziness, headache, nausea and vomiting, abdominal cramps, diaphoresis, bronchoconstriction, anaphylaxis.

Precautions: Coronary artery disease (may precipitate angina or MI), CHF, hepatic or renal impairment; seizure disorders, asthma, vascular disease.

Verapamil (Calan, Isoptin)

Class: Calcium channel blocker, antiarrhythmic, class IV, antihypertensive.

Indications: PSVT (with narrow QRS and adequate BP) refractory to adenosine; rapid ventricular rates in A-fib, A-flutter, and MAT.

Adult Dose: 2.5–5.0 mg IV over 2 min; may give second dose, if needed, of 5–10 mg IV in 15–30 min, max dose 20 mg. An alternative second dose is 5 mg IV every 15 min, max dose 30 mg.

Contraindications: A-fib with Wolff-Parkinson-White syndrome, wide-complex tachycardia of uncertain origin, second- or third-degree AV block (unless a functioning pacemaker is in place), sick sinus syndrome, hypotension, severe CHF, cardiogenic shock, concurrent IV beta blocker, VT.

Side Effects: Hypotension, exacerbation of CHF with left ventricular dysfunction, bradycardia, AV block, constipation, peripheral edema, headache, dizziness, fatigue, paralytic ileus, hepatotoxicity.

Precautions: Concurrent oral beta blockers, CHF, impaired hepatic or renal function, myasthenia gravis, muscular dystrophy, hypertrophic cardiomyopathy with outflow tract obstruction; may decrease myocardial contractility. In geriatric patients administer slowly over 3 min.

Common Medication Formulas

Syringe: Amount to be drawn up	$$\frac{\text{Desired dose of drug} \times \text{Total volume}}{\text{Total dose of drug on hand}}$$
IV: Calculating gtt/min	$$\frac{\text{Volume to be infused} \times \text{Drop (gtt) factor}}{\text{Total time in minutes}}$$
IV: Calculating infusion rate (mg/min or mcg/min)	$$\frac{\text{Volume on hand} \times \text{gtt factor} \times \text{Desired dose}}{\text{Total dose of drug on hand}} = \text{gtt/min}$$ Example: Administer 2 mg/min of lidocaine. To prepare the infusion, mix 2 g (2000 mg) of lidocaine in 500 mL of D5W with a drip set of 60 gtt/mL. Calculate the infusion rate. $\frac{500 \text{ mL} \times 60 \text{ gtt/mL} \times 2 \text{ mg}}{2000 \text{ mg}} = 30 \text{ gtt/min}$
IV: Rate of an existing IV	1. Count drops (gtt)/min and multiply by 60 min. 2. Divide result by the drop (gtt) factor being used.

IV Fluid Drip Rate Table (gtt/min)

Rate: (mL/hr) →	TKO	50	75	100	125	150	175	200	250
10 gtt/mL set	5	8	13	17	21	25	29	33	42
12 gtt/mL set	6	10	15	20	25	30	35	40	50
15 gtt/mL set	8	13	19	25	31	37	44	50	62
20 gtt/mL set	10	17	25	33	42	50	58	67	83
60 gtt/mL set	30	50	75	100	125	150	175	200	250

Universal Formula—Figure Out Drip Rates and Drug Amounts

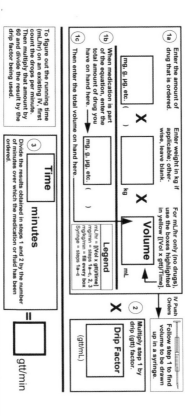

1a Enter the amount of drug that is ordered.

| mg, g, µg, etc. ( ) | × | Enter weight in kg if applicable; otherwise, leave blank. kg | × | For mL/hr only (no drugs), use the boxes highlighted in yellow [(IVol x gtt/Time)]. Volume mL |

1b When medication is part of the equation, enter the total amount of drug you have on hand here. → mg, g, µg, etc. ( )

1c Then enter the total volume on hand here.

Legend
mL/hr = [(IVol x gtt)/time]
mg/min = steps 1a–c, 2, 3
mcg/min = steps 1a–c
Syringe = fill every box

2 IV Push Orders
Follow step 1 to find volume to be drawn up in a syringe.
Multiply step 1 by drip (gtt) factor.

Drip Factor (gtt/mL)

3 Time minutes
Divide the results obtained in steps 1 and 2 by the number of minutes over which the medication or fluid has been ordered.

= gtt/min

To figure out the running time (mL/hr) on an existing IV, first count the drops per minute. Then multiply that amount by 60 and divide the result by the drip factor being used.

Note: The abbreviation mcg (microgram) means the same as µg (used in the above formula); mcg is used most commonly to prevent medication errors.

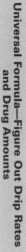

Emergency Medical Skills

Defibrillation

Indications: Ventricular fibrillation or pulseless VT.

Energy Levels: Use an adult biphasic energy level at 120–200 J (use the manufacturer's device-specific energy level) or deliver 360 J for a monophasic energy level. Continue at a biphasic energy level of 120–200 J for further shocks or a monophasic energy level of 360 J.

Application: Dry moisture off skin; shave excessive hair, if necessary. Use remote adhesive pads or handheld paddles. Always use a conducting gel with paddles and apply firm pressure (15–25 pounds per paddle) to the chest to ensure good skin contact.

Methods: Manual or automated.

Precautions: Place pads or paddles several inches away from an implanted pacemaker or ICD.

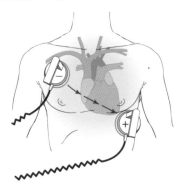

Placement of paddles for defibrillation

♥ **Clinical Tip:** Defibrillation may be used on infants younger than 1 year old and on children (1 yr to puberty). Always use pediatric pads or paddles and follow pediatric protocols.

Manual Defibrillation

A manual defibrillator is used to restore a normal heart rhythm. For a patient experiencing sudden cardiac arrest, first assess for responsiveness, respiration, and pulse. Begin CPR. Verify that the rhythm is either VF or pulseless VT, and then manually deliver an electric shock to the heart.

Procedure

1. Verify that the patient is in cardiac arrest, with no pulse or respiration. Have someone provide CPR while the defibrillator is obtained and placed next to the patient or left on the crash cart.
2. Turn on the defibrillator; verify that all cables are connected.
3. Turn "lead select" to "paddles" or "defibrillator."
4. Pads: Place in locations specified for paddles. Roll pads on from top to bottom edges to prevent air pockets. Paddles: Use conducting gel or gel pads and place on the apex (lower left chest, midaxillary) and sternum (right of sternum, midclavicular).
5. Remove oxygen away from patient and immediate vicinity.
6. Select the initial energy level for an adult to a biphasic energy level of 120–200 J (use the manufacturer's device-specific energy levels) or a monophasic energy level of 360 J.
7. Verify rhythm as VF or pulseless VT.
8. Say, "Charging defibrillator, stand clear!"
9. Charge the defibrillator.
10. Say, "I'm going to shock on three. One, I'm clear; two, you're clear; three, everybody's clear." Perform a visual sweep to ensure all rescue personnel are clear of the patient, bed, and equipment and oxygen is removed.
11. Discharge the defibrillator, reassess the rhythm, and refer to appropriate advanced cardiac life support protocol.

Automated External Defibrillator

An automated external defibrillator (AED) is a small, lightweight device used by both professionals and laypersons to assess heart rhythm by computer analysis. Using voice and visual prompts, it administers an electric shock, if necessary, to restore a normal rhythm in patients with sudden cardiac arrest. A shock is administered only if the rhythm detected is VF or pulseless VT. Automated external defibrillators are available from medical device manufacturers and local pharmacies. Although the AEDs all operate in basically the same way, external features vary from model to model. Be sure to follow the manufacturer's recommendations.

Indications: Ventricular fibrillation or pulseless VT in adults, children, and infants.

Dose: The AED will automatically select the energy dose for each defibrillation. Some devices are equipped with pediatric systems that include a pad–cable system or a key to reduce the delivered energy to a suitable dose for children.

Procedure

1. Verify that the patient is in cardiac arrest, with no pulse or respiration. Have someone provide CPR while the AED is obtained and placed next to the patient.
2. Power on the AED. Follow the voice prompts and visual messages.
3. Open the package of adhesive electrode pads and attach pads to the patient's bare chest.
4. Use adult pads for an adult and child pads for a child. If there are no child pads available, you may use adult pads on a child, but be sure the pads do not touch.
5. Attach one pad to the right sternal border (superior-anterior right chest) and place the second pad over the left apex (inferior-lateral left chest). Alternatively, follow the diagrams on each of the AED electrodes.
6. Connect the pad cables to the AED.
7. Clear the patient and stop CPR. Remove oxygen, if applicable.
8. The AED may automatically analyze the patient's rhythm or may be equipped with an "analyze" button.
9. If a shock is advised, say, "I'm going to shock on three. One, I'm clear; two, you're clear; three, everybody's clear." Perform a visual sweep to ensure rescue personnel are not touching the patient or equipment. Remove oxygen, if applicable. Press the shock button.
10. Once the shock is delivered, continue CPR beginning with chest compression.
11. After about 2 minutes of CPR, the AED will prompt you with further verbal and visual cues.

♥ **Clinical Tip:** A fully automated AED analyzes the rhythm and delivers a shock, if one is indicated, without operator intervention once the pads are applied to the patient.

♥ **Clinical Tip:** A semiautomated AED analyzes the rhythm and tells the operator that a shock is indicated. If it is, the operator initiates the shock by pushing the shock button.

Cardioversion (Synchronized)

Indications: Unstable tachycardias (50 bpm with a perfusing rhythm). The patient may present with an altered LOC, dizziness, chest pain, or hypotension.

Energy Levels: Regular narrow QRS complex tachycardias (supraventricular tachyarrhythmia)—generally requires less energy, 50 to 100 J either biphasic or monophasic is often sufficient; narrow irregular rhythm (atrial fibrillation)—120 to 200 J biphasic or 200 J monophasic. If the initial cardioversion shock fails, the energy should be increased in a stepwise fashion. Regular wide QRS complex tachycardias (monomorphic ventricular tachycardia)—responds well to biphasic or monophasic initial energies of 100 J. If there is no response to the first shock, it may be reasonable to increase the dose in stepwise fashion. Synchronized cardioversion must not be used for treatment of VF because the device is unlikely to sense a QRS wave and thus a shock may not be delivered. Synchronized cardioversion should also not be used for pulseless VT or polymorphic VT (irregular VT). These rhythms require delivery of high-energy unsynchronized shocks (i.e., defibrillation doses).

Application: Use remote adhesive pads or handheld paddles. Always use a conducting gel with paddles. For conscious patients, explain the procedure and use medication for sedation and analgesia. Consider 2.5–5.0 mg midazolam **(Versed),** or 5.0 mg diazepam **(Valium),** or 1–2 mcg/kg/min fentanyl IV, or anesthesia, if available.

Methods: Remove oxygen, if applicable. Place defibrillator in synchronized (sync) mode. Observe marker on R wave to confirm proper synchronization. Charge to appropriate level. Say, "I'm going to shock on three. One, I'm clear; two, you're clear; three, everybody's clear." Perform a visual sweep and ensure that oxygen is removed. Press and hold shock button until shock is delivered. If using paddles, press

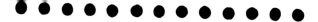

and hold both discharge buttons simultaneously until shock is delivered. Reassess the patient and treat according to the appropriate advanced cardiac life support protocol.

Precautions: Reactivate the "sync" mode after each attempted cardioversion; defibrillators default to the unsynchronized mode. Place pads or paddles several inches away from an implanted pacemaker or implantable cardioverter-defibrillator (ICD).

♥ **Clinical Tip:** The "sync" mode delivers energy synchronizing with the timing of the QRS complex to avoid stimulation during the refractory, or vulnerable, period of the cardiac cycle when a shock could potentially produce VF.

Transcutaneous Pacing

Indications: A temporizing measure for symptomatic bradycardia (with a pulse) unresponsive to atropine, bradycardia with ventricular escape rhythms, symptomatic second-degree AV block type II, or third-degree AV block.

Pacing Modes: *Demand-mode (synchronous)* pacemakers sense the patient's heart rate and pace only when the heart rate falls below the level set by the clinician. *Fixed-mode (asynchronous)* pacemakers cannot sense the heart rate and always operate at the rate set by the clinician. Rate selections vary between 30 and 180 bpm. Output is adjustable between 0 and 200 mA. Pulse duration varies from 20–40 ms.

Application: Pacemaker pads work most effectively if placed in an anterior-posterior position on the patient.

Contraindications: Not effective in VF, pulseless VT, or asystole.

Side Effects: Chest muscle contraction, burns, and chest discomfort.

Precautions: Make sure pads have good skin contact to achieve capture and avoid burns.

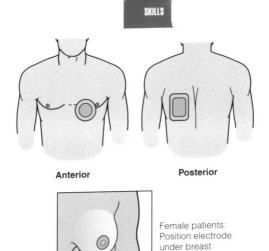

Anterior

Posterior

Female patients:
Position electrode
under breast

Placement of anterior-posterior pacemaker pads.

Carotid Sinus Massage (Vagal Maneuver)

Indications: Can increase vagal nerve stimulation and slow SVT, or even convert SVT to NSR, without severe hemodynamic compromise. **Should be performed only by qualified physicians due to the risk for stroke.**

Method: Place the patient in a supine position, head tilted to either side with the neck hyperextended. Place your index and middle fingers over the carotid artery just below the angle of the jaw, as high on the neck as possible. Massage the artery for 5–10 sec by pressing it firmly against the vertebral column and rubbing.

Contraindications: Unequal carotid pulses, carotid bruits, cervical spine injury, or history of cerebrovascular accident or carotid atherosclerosis.

Side Effects: Slow HR or AV block, PVCs, VT, VF, syncope, seizure, hypotension, nausea or vomiting, stroke.

Precautions: Be sure the patient is receiving oxygen and an IV is in place. Never massage both arteries simultaneously. Resuscitation equipment must be readily available.

♥ **Clinical Tip:** Performed only by qualified physicians. Each carotid artery should be palpated and auscultated before the procedure to evaluate for contraindications to carotid sinus massage.

♥ **Clinical Tip:** Alternate vagal maneuvers include encouraging the patient to cough, bear down, blow through an obstructed straw, place ice to the face, or hold his or her breath.

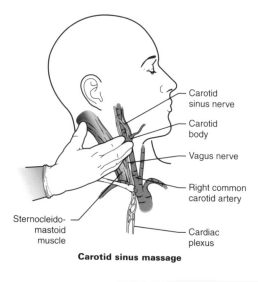

Carotid sinus nerve

Carotid body

Vagus nerve

Right common carotid artery

Cardiac plexus

Sternocleido-mastoid muscle

Carotid sinus massage

SKILLS

Healthcare Provider Guidelines for CPR

CPR Method	Compression/ Ventilation Ratio	Rate of Compressions (min)	Depth of Compressions	Pulse Check (artery)	Hand Position for Compressions
Adult, 1 rescuer	30:2	100–120	At least 2.0 in (5 cm)	Carotid	Heels of 2 hands on lower half of the sternum
Adult, 2 rescuers	30:2	100–120	At least 2.0 in (5 cm)	Carotid	Heels of 2 hands on lower half of the sternum
Child, 1 rescuer	30:2	100–120	At least ⅓ depth of chest (about 2.0 in [5 cm])	Carotid or femoral	Heel of 1 or 2 hands on lower half of the sternum between nipple line
Child, 2 rescuers	15:2	100–120	At least ⅓ depth of chest (about 2.0 in [5 cm])	Carotid or femoral	Heel of 1 or 2 hands over center of chest between nipple line
Infant, 1 rescuer	30:2	100–120	At least ⅓ depth of chest (about 1.5 in [4 cm])	Brachial	2 fingers over center of chest, just below nipple line.
Infant, 2 rescuers	15:2	100–120	At least ⅓ depth of chest (about 1.5 in [4 cm])	Brachial	2-thumbs-encircling-hands technique over center of chest, just below nipple line

CPR: Adult (Age of puberty or older)

1. Ensure that the scene is safe. **Check for unresponsiveness.** Gently tap the person's shoulder. Ask, "Are you OK?"

2. Simultaneously assess the person's breathing and pulse.
   - **Check for breathing.** Is the breathing normal, no breathing, or abnormal (only agonal gasps)?
   - **Assess the carotid pulse and look for other signs of circulation (no more than 10 sec).** If signs of circulation are present but the person is still not breathing, give rescue breaths at the rate of 10–12 breaths/min (1 breath every 5–6 sec).

3. **In a sudden collapse, if you are alone and there is no response with no breathing, abnormal breathing (only agonal gasps), and no pulse, summon help, call a code, or phone 911 and get an automated external defibrillator (AED), if available.** Send a second rescuer, if available, for help.

4. **Position the person supine** on a hard, flat surface.

5. If a pulse and signs of circulation are not present, **begin chest compressions.**
   - Place the heel of one hand on the center of the chest over the lower half of the sternum; place the heel of your other hand over the first.
   Firmly compress the chest at least 2.0 in (5 cm). Push hard and fast. Give 30 compressions. Compress at a rate of 100–120/min. Ensure complete chest recoil after each compression. Avoid leaning on the chest between compressions.

6. If the person is not breathing, begin rescue breaths. Open the airway by the head tilt–chin lift method or, if spinal injury is suspected, use the jaw thrust method, if possible.

7. Using a face mask or barrier device, give 2 breaths (1 sec each) with sufficient volume to cause the chest to rise. Do not overventilate. Note: If the chest does not rise, reposition the head, chin, and jaw, and give 2 more breaths. If the chest still does not rise, follow instructions for unconscious adult with an obstructed airway.

8. Continue to give 30 compressions followed by 2 breaths until an AED arrives. If an AED is unavailable, continue to give 30 compressions followed by 2 breaths.

CPR

9. If circulation resumes but breathing does not resume or is inadequate, continue rescue breathing at 10–12 breaths/min (1 breath every 5–6 sec).
10. If adequate breathing and circulation resume, place the person in the recovery position and monitor until help arrives.

♥ **Clinical Tip:** Chest compressions should be interrupted infrequently and for no longer than 10 seconds. Pulse checks, even to determine return of spontaneous circulation (ROSC), should be minimized during resuscitation.

♥ **Clinical Tip:** When two rescuers are available, give cycles of 30 compressions and 2 breaths for adult CPR. After every fifth cycle (2 min) rescuers should switch roles to minimize rescuer fatigue because compression rates and/or depth may become inadequate due to recognized or unrecognized fatigue. The switch should be accomplished in less than 5 sec. If available, a bag-valve-mask device can be used with two-rescuer CPR.

CPR: Child (1 yr to age of puberty)

1. Ensure that the scene is safe. Check for unresponsiveness. Gently tap child's shoulder. Ask, "Are you okay?"
2. Simultaneously assess the child's breathing and pulse.
   - **Check for breathing.** Is the breathing normal, no breathing, or abnormal (only agonal gasps)?
   - **Assess the carotid pulse and look for other signs of circulation (no more than 10 sec).** If signs of circulation are present but the child is still not breathing, give rescue breaths at the rate of 12–20 breaths/min (1 breath every 3–5 sec).
3. If there is no response with no breathing or abnormal breathing (only agonal gasps), send a second rescuer, if available, for help and to get an AED, if available.
4. If you are alone, begin the steps for CPR.
5. Position the child supine on a hard, flat surface.
6. If a pulse and signs of circulation are not present, begin chest compressions.
   - **One hand:** Place the heel of one hand on the center of the chest over the lower half of the sternum.

- ■ **Two hands:** Place the heel of one hand on the center of the chest over the lower half of the sternum; place the heel of your other hand over the first.

Firmly compress the chest at least one third the depth of the chest (at least 2.0 in [5 cm]). Push hard and fast. Give 30 compressions. Compress at a rate of 100–120/min. Ensure complete chest recoil after each compression. Avoid leaning on the chest between compressions.

7. If the child is not breathing, **begin rescue breaths.** Open the airway by the head tilt–chin lift method or, if spinal injury is suspected, use the jaw thrust method, if possible.

8. Using a face mask or barrier device, **give 2 breaths (1 sec each) with sufficient volume to cause the chest to rise. Do not overventilate.** Note: If the chest does not rise, reposition the head, chin, and jaw, and give 2 more breaths. **If the chest still does not rise, follow instructions for unconscious child with an obstructed airway.**

9. **Continue cycles of 30 compressions followed by 2 breaths.** After the fifth cycle of 30:2 (2 min), if you are still alone and no signs of circulation are present, **summon help, call a code, or phone 911 and get an AED, if available.**

10. If circulation is still not present, continue CPR, starting with chest compressions until an AED is available. If an AED is unavailable, continue to give 30 compressions followed by 2 breaths.

11. If circulation resumes but breathing does not resume or is inadequate, continue rescue breathing at 12–20 breaths/min.

12. If adequate breathing and circulation resume, place the child in the recovery position and monitor until help arrives.

♥ **Clinical Tip:** If you are alone and know a child or infant has had a sudden collapse because of heart failure, request immediate help including an AED. Do not delay defibrillation.

♥ **Clinical Tip:** When two rescuers are available, give cycles of 15 compressions and 2 breaths for child CPR.

CPR

CPR: Infant (Younger than 1 yr)

1. Ensure that the scene is safe. Check for unresponsiveness. Gently rub the infant's back or tap the feet.
2. Simultaneously assess the infant's breathing and pulse.
   - **Check for breathing.** Is the breathing normal, no breathing, or abnormal (only agonal gasps)?
   - **Assess the brachial pulse and look for other signs of circulation (no more than 10 sec).** If signs of circulation are present but the child is still not breathing, give rescue breaths at the rate of 12–20 breaths/min (1 breath every 3–5 sec).
3. If there is no response with no breathing or abnormal breathing (only agonal gasps), send a second rescuer, if available, for help and an AED, if available.
4. If you are alone, begin the steps for CPR.
5. Position the infant supine on a hard, flat surface.
6. If a pulse and signs of circulation are not present, **begin chest compressions.**
   - Place two fingers of one hand over the center of the chest just below the nipple line.
   Firmly compress the chest at least one third the depth of the chest (at least 1.5 in [4 cm]). Push hard and fast. Give 30 compressions. Compress at a rate of 100–120/min. Ensure complete chest recoil after each compression. Avoid leaning on the chest between compressions.
7. If the infant is not breathing, **begin rescue breaths.** Open the airway by the head tilt–chin lift method or, if spinal injury is suspected, use the jaw thrust method, if possible.
8. Using a face mask or barrier device, **give 2 breaths (1 sec each) with sufficient volume to cause the chest to rise. Do not overventilate.** Note: If the chest does not rise, reposition the head, chin, and jaw, and give 2 more breaths. **If the chest still does not rise, follow instructions for unconscious infant with an obstructed airway.**
9. **Continue to give 30 compressions followed by 2 breaths.** After the fifth cycle of 30:2 (2 min), if you are still alone and no signs of circulation are present, **summon help, call a code, or phone 911 and get an AED, if available.**
10. If circulation is still not present, continue CPR until the AED is available. If an AED is unavailable, continue to give 30 compressions followed by 2 breaths.

11. If circulation resumes but breathing does not resume or is inadequate, continue rescue breathing at 12–20 breaths/min.
12. If adequate breathing and circulation resume, place the infant in the recovery position and monitor until help arrives.

♥ **Clinical Tip:** When two rescuers are available, give cycles of 15 compressions and 2 breaths for infant CPR. Use the two-thumbs-encircling-hands technique for chest compressions. If available, a bag-valve-mask device can be used with two-person CPR.

Obstructed Airway: Conscious Adult or Child (1 yr or older)

Clinical Presentation

- Grabbing at the throat with one or both hands
- Inability to speak; high-pitched crowing sounds
- Wheezing, gagging, ineffective coughing
  1. Determine that the airway is obstructed. Ask, "Are you choking? Can you speak?"
  2. Let the person know you are going to help.
  3. Stand behind the choking person and wrap your arms around the person's waist. For someone who is obese or pregnant, wrap your arms around the chest.
  4. Make a fist. Place the thumb side of your fist in middle of the person's abdomen, just above the navel. Locate the middle of the sternum for obese or pregnant persons.
  5. Grasp your fist with your other hand.
  6. Press your fist abruptly into the person's abdomen using an upward, inward thrust. Use a straight chest thrust back for someone who is obese or pregnant.
  7. Continue abdominal or chest thrusts until the object is dislodged or the person loses consciousness.
  8. If the person loses consciousness, treat as an unconscious adult or a child with an obstructed airway.

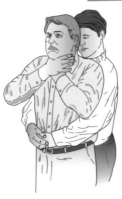

Abdominal thrusts for adult or child

Obstructed Airway: Conscious Infant (younger than 1 yr)

Clinical Presentation

- Inability to breathe or cry
- High-pitched crowing sounds
- Sudden wheezing or noisy breathing
  1. Determine that the airway is obstructed. Notice if air exchange is poor or does not occur.
  2. Lay the infant down on your forearm, supporting the jaw between your thumb and index finger and supporting the chest with your hand and forearm.
  3. Using your thigh or lap for support, keep the infant's head lower than the body.
  4. Give five quick, forceful slaps between the shoulder blades with the heel of your hand.
  5. Turn the infant over to be face up on your other arm. Using your thigh or lap for support, keep the infant's head lower than the body.

136

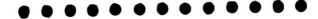

6. Place two fingers of one hand over the center of the chest just below the nipple line.
7. Give five quick thrusts downward, depressing the chest by ⅓ (1.5 in) its depth each time.
8. Continue the sequence of five back slaps and five chest thrusts until the object is dislodged or the infant loses consciousness. If the infant loses consciousness, treat as an unconscious infant with an obstructed airway.

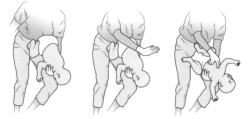

Back blows and chest thrusts for infant

Obstructed Airway: Unconscious Adult (Age of puberty or older)

Clinical Presentation

- Failure to breathe, cyanosis
- Inability to move air into lungs with rescue breaths
  1. Ensure that the scene is safe. **Check for unresponsiveness.** Gently tap the person's shoulder. Ask, "Are you OK?"
  2. Simultaneously assess the person's breathing and pulse.
     - **Check for breathing.** Is the breathing normal, no breathing, or abnormal (only agonal gasps)?
     - **Assess the carotid pulse and look for other signs of circulation (no more than 10 sec).** If signs of circulation are present but the person is still not breathing, give rescue breaths at the rate of 10–12 breaths/min (1 breath every 5–6 sec).

CPR

3. **In a sudden collapse, if there is no response with no breathing or abnormal breathing (only agonal gasps) and you are alone, summon help, call a code, or phone 911 and get an automated external defibrillator (AED), if available.** Send a second rescuer, if available, for help.

4. **Position the person supine** on a hard, flat surface.

5. If a pulse and signs of circulation are not present, **begin chest compressions.**
   - Place the heel of one hand on the center of the chest over the lower half of the sternum; place the heel of your other hand over the first.
   Firmly compress the chest at least 2.0 in (5 cm). Push hard and fast. Give 30 compressions. Compress at a rate of at least 100–120/min. Ensure complete chest recoil after each compression. Avoid leaning on the chest between compressions.

6. If the person is not breathing, **begin rescue breaths.** Open the airway by the head tilt–chin lift method or, if spinal injury is suspected, use the jaw thrust method, if possible.

7. Using a face mask or barrier device, **give 2 breaths (1 sec each) with sufficient volume to cause the chest to rise. Do not overventilate.** If the chest does not rise, reposition the head, chin, and jaw, and give 2 more breaths. **If the chest still does not rise,** each time the airway is opened, look for an object in the person's mouth. **Only use a finger sweep to remove material you see obstructing the airway. Never perform a finger sweep if you do not see a foreign body in the airway.**

8. **Continue to give 30 compressions followed by opening the airway, looking for an object, and performing a finger sweep if object is visible, and then attempt to give 2 breaths.**

9. **Continue these cycles until an AED arrives.** If an AED is unavailable, continue to give 30 compressions followed by 2 breaths.

10. If circulation resumes but breathing does not resume or is inadequate, continue rescue breathing at 10–12 breaths/min (1 breath every 5–6 sec).

11. If adequate breathing and circulation resume, place the person in the recovery position and monitor until help arrives.

♥ **Clinical Tip:** An airway obstruction is successfully removed if you see and remove the object or feel air movement and see the chest rise when you give breaths.

Obstructed Airway: Unconscious Child (1 yr to age of puberty)

Clinical Presentation

- Failure to breathe, cyanosis
- Inability to move air into lungs with rescue breaths
  1. Ensure that the scene is safe. **Check for unresponsiveness.** Gently tap child's shoulder. Ask, "Are you okay?"
  2. Simultaneously assess the child's breathing and pulse.
     - Check for breathing. Is the breathing normal, no breathing, or abnormal (only agonal gasps)?
     - **Assess the carotid pulse and look for other signs of circulation (no more than 10 sec).** If signs of circulation are present but the child is still not breathing, give rescue breaths at the rate of 12–20 breaths/min (1 breath every 3–5 sec).
  3. If **there is no response with no breathing, and no pulse, abnormal breathing (only agonal gasps)**, send a second rescuer, if available, for help and an AED, if available.
  4. If you are alone, begin the steps for CPR.
  5. **Position the child supine** on a hard, flat surface.
  6. If a pulse and signs of circulation are not present, **begin chest compressions.**
     - **One hand:** Place the heel of one hand on the center of the chest over the lower half of the sternum.
     - **Two hands:** Place the heel of one hand on the center of the chest over the lower half of the sternum; place the heel of your other hand over the first.

     Firmly compress the chest at least one third the depth of the chest (at least 2.0 in). Push hard and fast. Give 30 compressions. Compress at a rate of at least 100–120/min. Ensure complete chest recoil after each compression. Avoid leaning on the chest between compressions.
  7. If the child is not breathing, **begin rescue breaths.** Open the airway by the head tilt–chin lift method or, if spinal injury is suspected, use the jaw thrust method, if possible.
  8. Using a face mask or barrier device, **give 2 breaths (1 sec each) with sufficient volume to cause the chest to rise. Do not overventilate.**

CPR

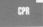

9. **If the chest does not rise, reposition the head, chin, and jaw, and give two more breaths.** Each time the airway is opened, look for an object in the child's mouth. **Only use a finger sweep to remove material you see obstructing the airway. Never perform a finger sweep if you do not see a foreign body in the airway.**

10. **Continue to give 30 compressions followed by opening the airway, looking for an object, and performing a finger sweep if object is visible, and then attempt to give 2 breaths.** After the fifth cycle of 30:2 (2 min), if you are still alone and no signs of circulation are present, summon help, call a code, or phone 911 and get an AED, if available.

11. If circulation is still not present, continue CPR until the AED is available. If an AED is unavailable, continue to give 30 compressions followed by 2 breaths. After each fifth cycle of 30:2 (2 min), recheck the pulse and look for other signs of circulation (no more than 10 sec).

12. If circulation resumes but breathing does not resume or is inadequate, continue rescue breathing at 12–20 breaths/min.

13. If adequate breathing and circulation resume, place the child in the recovery position and monitor until help arrives.

♥ **Clinical Tip:** Never perform a blind finger sweep.

Obstructed Airway: Unconscious Infant (younger than 1 yr)

Clinical Presentation

- Inability to breathe, high-pitched noises
- Inability to move air into lungs with rescue breaths
- Cyanosis
  1. Ensure that the scene is safe. **Check for unresponsiveness.** Gently rub the infant's back or tap the feet.
  2. Simultaneously assess the infant's breathing and pulse.
     - **Check for breathing.** Is the breathing normal, no breathing, or abnormal (only agonal gasps)?
     - **Assess the brachial pulse and look for other signs of circulation (no more than 10 sec).** If signs of circulation are present but the infant is still not breathing, give rescue breaths at the rate of 12–20 breaths/min (1 breath every 3–5 sec).

3. If **there is no response with no breathing, abnormal breathing (only agonal gasps)**, and no pulse, send a second rescuer, if available, for help.

4. If you are alone, begin the steps for CPR.

5. **Position the infant supine** on a hard, flat surface.

6. If a pulse and signs of circulation are not present, **begin chest compressions**.
   - Place two fingers of one hand over the center of the chest just below the nipple line.
   Firmly compress the chest at least one third the depth of the chest (at least 1.5 in [4 cm]). Push hard and fast. Give 30 compressions. Compress at a rate of at least 100–120/min. Ensure complete chest recoil after each compression. Avoid leaning on the chest between compressions.

7. If the infant is not breathing, **begin rescue breaths.** Open the airway by the head tilt–chin lift method or, if spinal injury is suspected, use the jaw thrust method, if possible.

8. Using a face mask or barrier device, **give 2 breaths (1 sec each) with sufficient volume to cause the chest to rise. Do not overventilate.**

9. **If the chest does not rise, reposition the head, chin, and jaw, and give two more breaths.** Each time the airway is opened, look for an object in the infant's mouth. **Only use a finger sweep to remove material you see obstructing the airway. Never perform a finger sweep if you do not see a foreign body in the airway.**

10. **Continue to give 30 compressions followed by opening the airway, looking for an object, and performing a finger sweep if object is visible, and then attempt to give 2 breaths.** After the fifth cycle of 30:2 (2 min), if you are still alone and no signs of circulation are present, **summon help, call a code, or phone 911 and get an AED, if available.**

11. If circulation is still not present, continue CPR until the AED is available. If an AED is unavailable, continue to give 30 compressions followed by 2 breaths.

12. If circulation resumes but breathing does not resume or is inadequate, continue rescue breathing at 12–20 breaths/min.

13. If adequate breathing and circulation resume, place the infant in the recovery position and monitor until help arrives.

♥ **Clinical Tip:** When you open an infant's airway by the head tilt–chin lift method, do not overextend the head or the airway will become obstructed.

CPR

Opioid-Associated Life-Threatening Emergency (Adult)

Clinical Presentation

- Suspected Opioid Overdose
- Unresponsiveness
  1. Ensure that the scene is safe. **Check for unresponsiveness.** Gently tap the person's shoulder. Ask, "Are you OK?"
  2. **Simultaneously access the person's breathing and pulse.**
     - **Check for breathing.** Is the breathing normal, no breathing, or abnormal (only agonal gasps)?
     - **Assess the carotid pulse and look for other signs of circulation (no more than 10 sec).** If signs of circulation are present but the person is still not breathing, give rescue breaths at the rate of 10–12 breaths/min (1 breath every 5–6 sec).
  3. **In a sudden collapse, if you are alone and there is no response with no breathing or abnormal breathing (only agonal gasps) and no pulse, summon help, call a code, or phone 911 and get an automated external defibrillator (AED) and naloxone, if available.** Send a second rescuer, if available, for help.
  4. **Position the person supine** on a hard, flat surface.
  5. If a pulse and signs of circulation are not present, **begin chest compressions.**
     - Place the heel of one hand on the center of the chest over the lower half of the breastbone; place the heel of your other hand over the first.

     Firmly compress the chest at least 2.0 in. Push hard and fast. Give 30 compressions. Compress at a rate of 100–120/min. Ensure complete chest recoil after each compression. Avoid leaning on the chest between compressions.
  6. If the person is not breathing, begin rescue breaths. Open the airway by the head tilt-chin lift method or, if spinal injury is suspected, use the jaw thrust method, if possible.

7. Using a face mask or barrier device, give 2 breaths (1 sec each) with sufficient volume to cause the chest to rise. Do not overventilate. Note: If the chest does not rise, reposition the head, chin, and jaw, and give 2 more breaths. If the chest still does not rise, follow instructions for unconscious adult with an obstructed airway.

8. Continue to give 30 compressions followed by 2 breaths until an **AED and naloxone** arrive.

9. Administer **naloxone** as soon as it is available. Give 2 mg intranasal or 0.4 mg IM. May repeat after 4 min.

10. Does the person respond?
    - **Yes:** If adequate breathing and circulation resume, place the person in the recovery position and monitor until help arrives. If the person stops responding, begin CPR and repeat naloxone.
    - **No:** Continue CPR and use the AED as soon as it is available. Continue until the person responds or until advanced help arrives.

CPR AND OBSTRUCTED AIRWAY POSITIONS

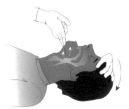

Head tilt–chin lift (adult or child)

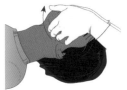

Jaw thrust maneuver

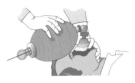

Bag-valve-mask

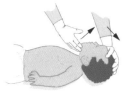

Head tilt–chin lift (infant)

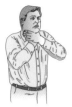

Universal choking sign

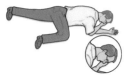

Recovery position.

ACLS: Ventricular Fibrillation (VF) or Pulseless Ventricular Tachycardia (VT)

Clinical Presentation
- Unresponsive state
- No respiration, pulse, or blood pressure (BP)
  1. Establish unresponsiveness with no respiration or pulse. Call for help.
  2. Begin CPR, provide oxygen, and attach AED or monitor-defibrillator when available without interrupting CPR.
  3. When device is attached, stop CPR and assess rhythm. If shock is advised when using an AED, **defibrillate following the AED voice/visual prompts.** If using a manual monitor-defibrillator and the rhythm is VF or pulseless VT, defibrillate at 120–200 J if using a biphasic defibrillator following manufacturer's device-specific energy levels if known, or 200 J if unknown, or defibrillate at 360 J if using a monophasic defibrillator.
  4. **Immediately resume CPR, beginning with compressions.** Provide five cycles (2 min) of uninterrupted CPR. During CPR, establish IV or intraosseous (IV/IO) access. Prepare vasopressor dose (epinephrine or vasopressin).
  5. Assess rhythm. **If the rhythm is shockable, follow AED voice/visual prompts or defibrillate at same or higher energy for biphasic manual defibrillator or at 360 J for a monophasic manual defibrillator.**
  6. Immediately **resume** CPR beginning with compressions and using five cycles of 30 compressions and 2 breaths.
  7. Consider insertion of an advanced airway (ET tube, LMA, King LT, or Combitube) if basic airway management is inadequate. **Once an advanced airway is in place, compressions should be uninterrupted at a rate of at least 100–120/min, and ventilations should be 10 breaths/min (1 breath every 6 sec).** Use waveform capnography to confirm and monitor ET tube placement.

8. Administer epinephrine 1 mg (10 mL of 1:10,000) by the IV/IO **method**; follow with 20-mL IV flush. Repeat every 3–5 min. If no IV/IO access is available, give 2.0–2.5 mg (1:1000) epinephrine diluted in 5–10 mL normal saline or sterile water and administer by endotracheal (ET) tube every 3–5 min until IV/IO access is available.

9. Continue CPR; check the rhythm every 2 min.

10. **If the rhythm is still shockable, defibrillate as in step 5.**

11. Immediately **resume** CPR; check the rhythm every 2 minutes.

Consider antiarrhythmics for shock-refractory VF or pulseless VT:

12. Administer amiodarone 300 mg IV/IO or lidocaine 1.0–1.5 mg/kg IV/IO. Lidocaine should only be used as an alternative if the patient is allergic to amiodarone or if amiodarone is unavailable.

13. Repeat antiarrhythmic therapy for shock-refractory VF or VT: amiodarone 150 mg IV/IO in 3–5 min (use only one time); or lidocaine 0.5–0.75 mg/kg IV/IO. Repeat lidocaine every 5–10 min, maximum dose 3 mg/kg. Lidocaine should only be used as an alternative if the patient is allergic to amiodarone or if amiodarone is unavailable.

14. Consider magnesium sulfate 1–2 g (2–4 mL of a 50% solution) diluted in 10 mL of D5W IV/IO, **given** over 1–2 min for cardiac arrest caused by hypomagnesemia or torsade de pointes.

♥ **Clinical Tip:** Do not delay defibrillation for a witnessed arrest. For an unwitnessed arrest with a down time greater than 4–5 min, perform 2 min of CPR before defibrillation.

♥ **Clinical Tip:** Airway must be secured and placement verified with observation of chest rise and auscultation of breath sounds plus a confirmatory device (exhaled CO_2 detector). Monitor tube for displacement during transport or whenever patient is moved.

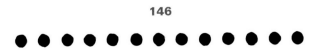

ACLS: Pulseless Electrical Activity (PEA)

Clinical Presentation
- Unresponsive state
- No respiration, pulse, or BP
- Identifiable organized electrical rhythm on monitor but no pulse
  1. Establish unresponsiveness with no respiration or pulse. Call for help.
  2. Begin CPR, provide oxygen, and attach manual monitor-defibrillator when available without interrupting CPR.
  3. When device is attached, stop CPR to assess rhythm. If organized rhythm noted on monitor, immediately resume CPR beginning with compressions. Establish IV/IO access.
  4. **During CPR, consider and treat possible causes:**
     - Hypokalemia/hyperkalemia
     - Hypothermia
     - Hypoxia
     - Hypovolemia
     - Hydrogen ion (acidosis)
     - Tension pneumothorax
     - Thrombosis, pulmonary
     - Thrombosis, coronary
     - Tamponade, cardiac
     - Toxins
  5. Continue CPR using five cycles of 30 compressions and 2 breaths; check the rhythm every 2 minutes.
  6. **Consider insertion of an advanced airway (ET tube, LMA, King LT, or Combitube) if basic airway management is inadequate.** After an advanced airway is in place, compressions should be uninterrupted at a rate of at least 100/min, and ventilations should be 8–10 breaths/min (1 breath every 6–8 sec). Use waveform capnography to confirm and monitor ET tube placement.
  7. If PEA persists, administer epinephrine 1 mg (10 mL of 1:10,000) by the IV/IO method; follow with 20-mL IV flush. Repeat every 3–5 min. If no IV/IO access is available, give 2.0–2.5 mg (1:1000) epinephrine diluted in 5–10 mL normal saline or sterile water and administer by endotracheal (ET) tube every 3–5 min until IV/IO access is available.
  8. Continue CPR; check the rhythm every 2 min.
  9. If the rhythm is shockable with no pulse, follow VF/VT protocol.

10. If the rhythm is not shockable with no pulse, resume CPR and repeat steps 4–8.

11. If a stable ECG rhythm returns with adequate breathing and circulation, monitor and reevaluate the patient.

♥ **Clinical Tip:** PEA is frequently caused by potentially reversible conditions and can be treated successfully if those conditions are identified and corrected easily.

ACLS: Asystole

Clinical Presentation

- Unresponsive state, no respiration, pulse, or BP
- ECG shows flat line; no electrical activity

1. Establish unresponsiveness with no respiration or pulse. Call for help.

2. Begin CPR, provide oxygen, and attach manual monitor-defibrillator when available without interrupting CPR.

3. When device is attached, stop CPR to assess rhythm. If no electrical activity (flat line or asystole) is noted on monitor, immediately resume CPR beginning with compressions. Establish IV/IO access.

4. **During CPR consider and treat possible causes:**

- Hypokalemia/hyperkalemia
- Hypovolemia
- Hypoxia
- Hypothermia
- Hydrogen ion (acidosis)
- Tension pneumothorax
- Thrombosis, pulmonary
- Thrombosis, coronary
- Tamponade, cardiac
- Toxins

5. Continue CPR beginning with compressions and using five cycles of 30 compressions and 2 breaths; check the rhythm every 2 min.

6. Consider insertion of an advanced airway (ET tube, LMA, King LT, or Combitube) if basic airway management is inadequate. **After an advanced airway is in place, compressions should be uninterrupted at a rate of 100–120/min, and ventilations should be 10 breaths/min (1 breath every 6 sec).** Use waveform capnography to confirm and monitor ET tube placement.

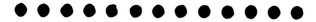

7. If asystole persists, administer epinephrine 1 mg (10 mL of 1:10,000) by the IV/IO method; follow with 20 mL IV flush. Repeat every 3–5 minutes. If no IV/IO access is available, give 2.0–2.5 mg (1:1,000) epinephrine diluted in 5–10 mL normal saline or sterile water and administer by endotracheal (ET) tube every 3–5 minutes until IV/IO access is available.

8. **Continue CPR; check the rhythm every 2 min.**

9. If the rhythm is shockable with no pulse, follow VF/VT protocol.

10. If the rhythm is not shockable with no pulse, resume CPR and repeat steps 4–8.

11. If asystole persists, consider whether proper resuscitation protocols were followed and reversible causes identified. If procedures were performed correctly, follow local criteria for terminating resuscitation efforts.

♥ **Clinical Tip:** Transcutaneous pacing is not recommended for asystolic cardiac arrest.

♥ **Clinical Tip:** Study local policy to learn established criteria for stopping resuscitation efforts.

ACLS: Acute Coronary Syndrome (ACS)

Clinical Presentation

- History of coronary artery disease, angina, or acute myocardial infarction (MI)
- Chest pain or discomfort
- Pain spreading to neck, shoulders, arms, jaw, or upper back
- Sudden unexplained shortness of breath, weakness, fatigue with or without chest pain/discomfort
- Associated nausea, diaphoresis, lightheadedness, fainting
  1. Establish responsiveness.
  2. Perform primary ABCD survey.
  3. Measure vital signs, including oxygen saturation.
  4. **Administer oxygen if oxygen saturation is <94%. Titrate to effect.**

5. **Administer aspirin 160–325 mg orally (PO)** if no history of aspirin allergy. Aspirin 81 mg (times 4 tablets) is commonly given. Chewing the tablet(s) is preferable; use nonenteric coated tablets for antiplatelet effect. Give within minutes of onset.

6. Start an IV and attach a cardiac monitor. Obtain a 12-lead ECG.

7. If the 12-lead ECG shows ST segment elevation, notify the attending physician. Begin the checklist for fibrinolytic therapy. If possible, prehospital providers should transport the patient to the closest facility with rapid coronary intervention capabilities.

8. **Administer nitroglycerin by the sublingual route 0.3–0.4 mg (1 tablet)**, repeated every 3–5 min for a total of three doses over a 15-min interval, or administer aerosol spray for 0.5–1.0 sec at 3–5 min intervals (provides 0.4 mg per dose) not to exceed three sprays in 15 min. **Nitroglycerin administration requires a systolic BP of 90 mm Hg or greater.**

9. Repeat nitroglycerin (see step 8) until chest pain is relieved, systolic BP falls below 90 mm Hg, or signs of ischemia or infarction are resolved.

10. If chest pain is not relieved by nitroglycerin, **administer morphine 2–4 mg IV (over 1–5 min)**. If symptoms are not resolved, administer 2–8 mg every 5–15 min if hemodynamically stable. Do not administer morphine if systolic BP is less than 90 mm Hg.

♥ **Clinical Tip:** Do not delay rapid transport to a cardiac catheterization laboratory for reperfusion. Consider fibrinolytic therapy within 30 minutes if a cardiac catheterization laboratory is not immediately available.

♥ **Clinical Tip:** Patients should not be given nitroglycerin if they have taken sildenafil (**Viagra**) or vardenafil (**Levitra**) in the last 24 hours or tadalafil (**Cialis**) within 48 hours. The use of nitroglycerin with these medications may cause irreversible hypotension.

♥ **Clinical Tip:** Nitroglycerin should be used with caution in patients with an inferior MI with possible right ventricular involvement. It is contraindicated with right ventricular MI, tachycardia, and bradycardia.

♥ **Clinical Tip:** Diabetic patients, elderly patients, and women frequently present with atypical symptoms (e.g., weakness, fatigue, complaints of indigestion).

ACLS: Bradycardia

Clinical Presentation

- Heart rate less than 50 bpm in symptomatic patient.
- Sinus bradycardia, junctional escape rhythm, or AV block
- Symptoms of chest discomfort/pain, lightheadedness, dizziness, dyspnea, tachypnea, presyncope, syncope.
- Signs of hypoxemia, hypotension, diaphoresis, altered mental status, congestive heart failure (CHF), shock

1. Establish responsiveness.
2. Perform primary ABCD survey.
3. Measure vital signs, including oxygen saturation.
4. Administer oxygen if oxygen saturation is <94%. Titrate to effect. Start an IV and attach cardiac monitor to identify rhythm.
5. Obtain a 12-lead ECG.
6. If the patient is stable and asymptomatic with a heart rate less than 50 bpm, monitor and observe for any changes.
7. If the patient is symptomatic with signs of poor perfusion, initiate treatment.
8. **Administer atropine 0.5 mg IV every 3–5 min**, maximum total dose 3 mg. In sinus bradycardia, junctional escape rhythm, or second-degree AV block Wenckebach/Mobitz type I, atropine is usually effective. In second-degree Mobitz type II or third-degree AV block, atropine is likely to be ineffective; prepare for transcutaneous pacing.
9. If the patient fails to respond to atropine in step 8, sedate and begin transcutaneous pacing (TCP) as a temporizing measure if IV access is not available. TCP is painful and will require sedation/analgesia in the conscious patient.
10. If the patient is hypotensive with severe bradycardia, or if TCP is unavailable or ineffective, initiate drug therapy with a **continuous dopamine infusion starting at 2–10 mcg/kg/min (chronotropic or heart rate dose)** and titrate to patient response. Mix 400 mg/250 mL in normal saline, lactated Ringer's solution, or D5W (1600 mcg/mL). An alternative may be an epinephrine infusion, 2–10 mcg/min IV (add 1 mg of 1:1000 in 500 mL normal saline and infuse at 1–5 mL/min). Seek expert consultation and prepare for transvenous pacing.

♥ **Clinical Tip:** If the patient has symptoms, do not delay transcutaneous pacing while waiting for atropine to take effect or for IV access.

♥ **Clinical Tip:** Use atropine with caution in a suspected acute MI; atropine may lead to rate-induced ischemia.

ACLS: Tachycardia—Unstable

Clinical Presentation

- Altered level of consciousness (LOC)
- Symptoms of shortness of breath, diaphoresis, weakness, fatigue, syncope or presyncope, chest discomfort or pain, palpitations
- Signs of hypotension, shock, congestive heart failure, ischemic ECG changes, poor peripheral perfusion
- Heart rate typically ≥150 bpm
  1. Establish responsiveness.
  2. Perform primary ABCD survey.
  3. Measure vital signs, including oxygen saturation.
  4. **Administer oxygen if oxygen saturation is <94%.** Titrate to effect. Start an IV and begin cardiac monitoring.
  5. Establish that serious signs and symptoms are related to the tachycardia.
  6. If the patient is **unstable and has symptoms** with a heart rate ≥150 bpm, prepare for immediate synchronized cardioversion (patients with a healthy heart are unlikely to be unstable if the ventricular rate is less than 150 bpm; however, patients with cardiac disease may be unstable with a heart rate less than 150 bpm). It is important to look at the patient's stability in addition to monitoring heart rate as criteria for cardioversion.
  7. Premedicate with a sedative plus an analgesic whenever possible.
  8. Place the defibrillator in synchronized (sync) mode.

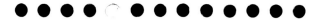

9. Administer synchronized cardioversion at:
- **Narrow regular rhythm (supraventricular tachyarrhythmia [SVT])**—generally requires less energy, 50 to 100 J either biphasic or monophasic is often sufficient; **narrow irregular rhythm (atrial fibrillation)**—120 to 200 J biphasic or 200 J monophasic. If the initial cardioversion shock fails, the energy should be increased in a stepwise fashion.
- **Wide regular rhythm (monomorphic ventricular tachycardia)**— usually responds well to biphasic or monophasic initial energies of 100 J. If there is no response to the first shock, it may be reasonable to increase the dose in a stepwise fashion.

10. If **a regular narrow complex tachycardia** is seen in an unstable patient, consider administering adenosine before cardioversion.
- **Adenosine**—6 mg IVP in the antecubital or other large vein given rapidly over 1–3 seconds followed by a 20-mL bolus of normal saline. If the rhythm has not converted in 1–2 min, repeat adenosine at 12 mg IVP. If the rhythm still does not convert, a third dose of 12 mg IVP may be given after another 1–2 min, maximum 30 mg.

11. If pulseless arrest develops, identify arrhythmia and follow algorithm for VF/VT, PEA, or asystole.

♥ **Clinical Tip:** Reactivate the "sync" mode before each attempted cardioversion.

♥ **Clinical Tip:** The "sync" mode delivers energy synchronizing with the timing of the QRS complex to avoid stimulation during the refractory, or vulnerable, period of the cardiac cycle when a shock could potentially produce VF.

♥ **Clinical Tip:** Synchronized cardioversion **must not be used** for treatment of VF because the device is unlikely to sense a QRS wave, and thus a shock may not be delivered. Synchronized cardioversion should also not be used for pulseless VT or polymorphic VT (irregular VT). These rhythms require delivery of high-energy unsynchronized shocks (i.e., defibrillation doses).

Narrow-Complex Tachycardia—Stable Regular Rhythm

Clinical Presentation
- No *serious* signs or symptoms related to the tachycardia
- Regular ECG rhythm
- QRS narrow (<0.12 sec)
- Heart rate typically ≥150 bpm
  1. Establish responsiveness.
  2. Perform primary ABCD survey.
  3. Measure vital signs, including oxygen saturation.
  4. **Administer oxygen if oxygen saturation is <94%.** Titrate to effect. Start an IV line, and attach cardiac monitor to identify rhythm. Obtain a 12-lead ECG.
  5. **Attempt vagal maneuvers** such as ice to the face (diving reflex), holding the breath while bearing down (Valsalva maneuver), or blowing through an obstructed straw.
  6. If rhythm has not converted to sinus rhythm, administer adenosine 6 mg IV in the antecubital or other large vein given rapidly over 1–3 sec followed by a 20-mL bolus of normal saline.
  7. If the rhythm has not converted in 1–2 min, repeat adenosine at 12 mg IV. If the rhythm still does not convert, a third dose of 12 mg IV may be given after another 1–2 min, maximum 30 mg.
  8. If the rhythm still does not convert, it may be atrial flutter, atrial tachycardia, multifocal atrial tachycardia, or junctional tachycardia. Consider rate control using diltiazem or beta blockers. Obtain expert consultation.
  9. If the rhythm converts, observe the patient and treat any recurrence with adenosine, diltiazem, or beta blockers. Obtain expert consultation.

♥ **Clinical Tip:** If the patient's condition becomes unstable during the tachycardia, perform immediate synchronized cardioversion.
♥ **Clinical Tip:** Use beta blockers with caution in patients with obstructive pulmonary disease or congestive heart failure. Avoid use in patients with bronchospastic disease.

Wide-Complex Tachycardia—Stable Regular Rhythm

Clinical Presentation

■ No *serious* signs and symptoms related to the tachycardia

■ Regular ECG rhythm

■ QRS wide (>0.12 sec)

■ Heart rate typically ≥150 bpm

1. Establish responsiveness.

2. Perform primary ABCD survey.

3. Measure vital signs, including oxygen saturation.

4. **Administer oxygen if oxygen saturation is <94%.** Titrate to effect. Start an IV, and attach cardiac monitor to identify rhythm. Obtain a 12-lead ECG.

5. If the arrhythmia is VT, administer amiodarone 150 mg IV/IO over 10 minutes. May repeat every 10 minutes and start infusion at 1 mg/min for 6 hours, followed by 0.5 mg/min for 18 hours. Do not exceed 2.2 g in 24 hours.

6. If the wide-complex tachycardia is regular, monomorphic, and suspected to be SVT with aberrancy, administer adenosine 6 mg IV in the antecubital or other large vein given rapidly over 1–3 seconds followed by a 20-mL bolus of normal saline.

7. If the rhythm transiently slows or converts to a sinus rhythm, it likely was SVT. However, if there was no effect after adenosine, the rhythm is likely monomorphic VT or atrial fibrillation with preexcitation and should be treated with amiodarone.

8. If pulseless arrest develops, identify arrhythmia and follow algorithm for VF/VT.

Immediate Post–Cardiac Arrest Care

Upon return of spontaneous circulation:

1. Provide oxygen to maintain oxygen saturation (94%–99% for optimal oxygenation. Avoid hyperoxygenation and oxygen toxicity.
2. Unless awake and alert, the patient may require an advanced airway and monitoring with waveform capnography.
   - Hyperventilation must be avoided.
   - Target end-tidal CO_2 (PET CO_2) should be 35–40 mm Hg, or $PaCO_2$ 40–45 mm Hg.
3. Monitor vital signs.
   - Systolic blood pressure should be maintained at 90 mm Hg or above, mean arterial pressure ≥65 mm Hg to optimize BP, cardiac output, and perfusion.
   - Treat hypotension.
     - If the systolic BP is <90 mm Hg, administer a 1- to 2-L fluid bolus of normal saline or lactated Ringer's.
     - If necessary, the patient may be treated with a vasopressor infusion: epinephrine, dopamine, or norepinephrine.
4. Consider and treat potentially reversible causes of cardiac arrest:
   - Hypokalemia/hyperkalemia
   - Hypovolemia
   - Hypoxia
   - Hypothermia
   - Hydrogen ion (acidosis)
   - Tension pneumothorax
   - Thrombosis, pulmonary
   - Thrombosis, coronary
   - Tamponade, cardiac
   - Toxins
5. Obtain a 12-lead ECG as soon as possible.
6. If the patient is comatose (lacking meaningful response to verbal commands):
   - Initiate Targeted Temperature Management (TTM) with a targeted temperature between 32°–36° C, selected and achieved, then maintained constantly for at least 24 hours.
7. If the patient rules in for an ST-elevation MI, or there is high suspicion for an acute MI:
   - Arrange for prompt transport to a cardiac catheterization laboratory for coronary reperfusion with possible percutaneous coronary intervention, maintaining hypothermia.

156

8. Maintain glycemic control.
   - Maintain blood glucose 144–180 mg/dL after arrest.
   - Avoid hypoglycemia.
9. Advanced critical care with development of a comprehensive plan of care should be provided to all survivors of cardiac arrest to optimize neurological, cardiopulmonary, and metabolic function.
   - Goal is return to patient's prearrest functional status.
   - Use of appropriate tools to establish prognosis for patients requiring continued advanced life support before determination to withdraw life support.

Stroke

Clinical Presentation
- Facial droop, arm or leg weakness/numbness, especially unilateral
- Difficulty speaking or understanding, confusion
- Sudden severe headache, visual disturbances, dizziness, loss of balance or coordination

The importance of rapid recognition of stroke symptoms, immediate activation of EMS, and rapid dispatch cannot be overemphasized.

EMS Response:
1. Support airway, breathing, and circulation.
   - Administer oxygen if needed (i.e., oxygen saturation <94%).
2. Perform prehospital stroke assessment.
   - Cincinnati Prehospital Stroke Scale.
3. Establish time when patient was last known to be normal or time of symptom onset if known.
4. Rapid transport: Triage to a center capable of providing acute stroke care if available.
5. Alert hospital.
   - Be sure hospital CT scan is functional.
6. Check patient's glucose level.

The following should be performed within first 60 min after patient has arrived at emergency department:

Immediate general assessment and stabilization within first 10 min of arrival:

1. Assess airway, breathing, circulation, and vital signs.
2. Administer oxygen if patient is hypoxemic.
3. Obtain IV access and blood samples.
4. Check glucose level.
   ■ Treat if indicated.
5. Perform initial neurological screening.
6. Activate stroke team.
7. Order emergent noncontrast CT scan or MRI of brain.
   ■ This is the most important test for a patient with a suspected acute stroke.
8. Obtain 12-lead ECG.

Immediate neurological assessment by stroke team or designee within first 25 min of arrival:

1. Review patient's history and perform general physical exam.
2. Establish time of symptom onset or last time patient was known to be normal.
3. Perform a neurological examination.
   ■ Use a stroke or neurological scale, such as the National Institutes of Health Stroke Scale (NIHSS) or Canadian Neurological Scale.
4. Interpret CT scan within 45 min of arrival.
5. Does CT scan show hemorrhage?

If CT scan does not show hemorrhage, perform the following within the first 45 min of arrival:

1. Review fibrinolytic inclusion, exclusion, and relative exclusion criteria.
2. Repeat neurological examination to determine whether patient's symptoms are improving/resolving or not.
3. If patient is a candidate for fibrinolytic therapy:
   ■ Review risks and benefits of fibrinolytic therapy with patient/family.
   ■ If patient/family agree, give rtPA within 60 min of arrival.
   ■ Do not give anticoagulants or antiplatelet treatment for 24 hours.
   ■ Begin post-rtPA stroke pathway.
   ■ Admit to stroke unit or intensive care unit.

- ■ Initiate supportive therapy.
- ■ Treat comorbidities.

4. If patient is not a candidate for fibrinolytic therapy:
   - ■ Administer aspirin (orally if the patient can swallow, or rectally if the patient has difficulty swallowing).
   - ■ Begin stroke pathway.
   - ■ Admit to stroke unit or intensive care unit.
   - ■ Initiate supportive therapy.
   - ■ Treat comorbidities.

If CT scan shows hemorrhage, perform the following within the first 45 minutes of arrival:

1. No aspirin, anticoagulation, or fibrinolytic therapy.
2. Consult neurologist or neurosurgeon.
   - ■ Consider transfer if such expertise is not available.
3. Initiate supportive therapy.
4. Begin stroke pathway within 60 min of arrival.
5. Admit to stroke unit or intensive care unit within 3 hours of arrival.
6. Treat comorbidities.

General Stroke Care

1. Begin stroke pathway.
2. Continue to support airway, breathing, and circulation.
   - ■ Maintain oxygen saturation 94%–99%.
3. Cardiac monitoring for first 24 hours or longer, if indicated.
4. Avoid intravenous D5W or excessive fluid loading.
5. Monitor blood pressure.
   - ■ Manage hypertension if systolic blood pressure is >220 mm Hg or diastolic blood pressure is >120 mm Hg.
6. Monitor blood glucose.
   - ■ Treat hyperglycemia.
7. Monitor temperature.
   - ■ Treat fever with acetaminophen.
8. Perform dysphagia screening/swallow evaluation.
9. Monitor for complications of stroke and fibrinolytic therapy (if administered).

Cincinnati Prehospital Stroke Scale

Facial droop: Have patient show teeth or smile.
- Normal—Both sides of face move equally well.
- Abnormal—One side of face does not move as well as the other side.

Arm drift: Have patient close eyes and hold both arms straight out with palms up for 10 sec
- Normal—Both arms move the same or do not move at all.
- Abnormal—One arm does not move or drifts down lower than the other.

Speech: Have the patient say "You can't teach an old dog new tricks."
- Normal—Patient uses correct words with no slurring.
- Abnormal—Patient slurs words, uses inappropriate words, or is unable to speak.

Note: The presence of a single abnormality has a sensitivity of 59% and a specificity of 89% when scored by prehospital providers.

Glasgow Coma Scale

Observation	Response	Score
Eye response	• Opens spontaneously	4
	• Opens to verbal commands	3
	• Opens to pain	2
	• No response	1
Best verbal response	• Alert and oriented	5
	• Disoriented but converses	4
	• Uses inappropriate words	3
	• Makes incomprehensible sounds	2
	• No response	1
Best motor response	• Reacts to verbal commands	6
	• Reacts to localized pain	5
	• Withdraws from pain	4
	• Abnormal flexion	3
	• Abnormal extension	2
	• No response	1
Total score	Normal	15

Score can range from 3 (lowest neurological function) to 15 (highest function).
Score 14–15: Mild dysfunction
Score 11–13: Moderate to severe dysfunction
Score ≤10: Severe dysfunction

160

PALS: Ventricular Fibrillation (VF) or Pulseless Ventricular Tachycardia (VT)

Clinical Presentation

- Pediatric patient
- Unresponsive state
- No respirations or only agonal respirations
- No pulse
- VF or pulseless VT on ECG monitor
  1. Establish unresponsiveness with no respirations or only agonal respirations with no pulse. Call for help.
  2. **Begin CPR. Provide oxygen as soon as available.**
  3. Attach an AED or monitor-defibrillator as soon as available without interrupting CPR. **Use pediatric pads or paddles if available and indicated.**
  4. When device is attached, stop CPR, check rhythm, and **defibrillate,** if advised.
     - If using an AED and shock is advised, defibrillate following AED voice/visual prompts. Attach monitor-defibrillator as soon as available to assess rhythm.
     - If using a manual monitor-defibrillator, assess the rhythm. If rhythm is VF or pulseless VT, defibrillate at 2 J/kg using a biphasic or monophasic defibrillator.
  5. Immediately resume CPR, beginning with compressions.
     - Two-rescuer CPR: Cycles of 15 compressions followed by 2 breaths.
     - Provide 2 min of uninterrupted CPR.
  6. During CPR, establish IV or IO access.
     - Prepare vasopressor dose (epinephrine).
  7. Stop CPR and assess rhythm. **Defibrillate** if rhythm remains shockable; follow AED voice/visual prompts or defibrillate at 4 J/kg.
  8. Immediately resume CPR, beginning with compressions, providing 2 min of uninterrupted CPR.

9. Administer epinephrine 0.01 mg/kg IV/IO (0.1 mL/kg of 1:10,000); follow with 20-mL IV flush.
   - Repeat every 3–5 min as needed.
   - If no IV/IO access is available and the patient has an endotracheal (ET) tube in place, inject 0.1 mg/kg (0.1 mL/kg of 1:1,000) epinephrine directly into ET tube followed by a 5-mL saline flush.
   - Follow ET drug administration with ventilations to disperse drug into small airways for absorption into pulmonary vasculature.
10. Insert an advanced airway (ET tube) if basic airway management is inadequate.
    - Confirm tube placement without interrupting CPR.
    - After correct placement is confirmed, deliver uninterrupted chest compressions at a rate of 100–120/min for 2 min and deliver 10 breaths/min at a rate of 1 breath every 6 sec.
11. Continue CPR and check the rhythm every 2 min.
12. If rhythm remains shockable, **defibrillate.** Follow AED voice/visual prompts or defibrillate at 4 J/kg.
    - May increase energy with subsequent shocks, if needed, up to a maximum of 10 J/kg or adult maximum energy dose.
13. Immediately resume CPR beginning with compressions. Check the rhythm every 2 min.
14. **Consider antiarrhythmic drugs for shock-refractory VF or pulseless VT:**
    - Administer amiodarone 5 mg/kg IV/IO, or lidocaine 1 mg/kg IV/IO if amiodarone is not available.
    - May repeat amiodarone 5 mg/kg IV/IO up to 2 times for shock-refractory VF or VT to a maximum of 15 mg/kg.
    - If the arrhythmia is torsade de pointes, consider magnesium sulfate 25–50 mg/kg IV/IO (maximum dose 2 g) bolus.
15. During CPR, consider and treat potentially reversible causes:
    - Hypoxia or ventilation problems
    - Hypovolemia
    - Hypothermia
    - Hypoglycemia
    - Hydrogen ion (acidosis)
    - Hypokalemia/hyperkalemia
    - Trauma (hypovolemia, increased ICP)
    - Tension pneumothorax
    - Tamponade (cardiac)
    - Toxins
    - Thrombosis (pulmonary or coronary)

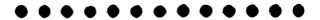

16. If rhythm changes to asystole or PEA, follow asystole or PEA protocol.

17. If rhythm converts to a stable ECG rhythm with return of spontaneous circulation, monitor and reevaluate the patient. Arrange for transport to a critical care unit. The patient will need a comprehensive plan of care.

♥ **Clinical Tip:** In infants and young children, the cause of cardiac arrest is more likely to be progressive respiratory failure or shock leading to an asphyxia arrest, rather than cardiac disease. Early recognition and management of impending respiratory failure may prevent cardiac arrest.

♥ **Clinical Tip:** Signs of impending respiratory failure include tachypnea, nasal flaring, intercostal and sternal retractions, grunting, and seesaw breathing.

♥ **Clinical Tip:** Use infant defibrillation pads or paddles for infants weighing <10 kg. Use adult pads or paddles for infants/children weighing ≥10 kg.

♥ **Clinical Tip:** Advanced airway must be secured and placement verified with observation of bilateral chest expansion, auscultation of bilateral breath sounds and lack of epigastric sounds, plus a confirmatory device (exhaled CO_2 detector). Use continuous waveform capnography if available. If not available, use a colorimetric CO_2 detector. Monitor tube for displacement during transport or whenever the patient is moved.

♥ **Clinical Tip:** After an advanced airway is in place, chest compressions should be delivered continuously without pausing for ventilations. A breath is delivered every 6–8 seconds without regard to the phase of chest compressions (downstroke vs. upstroke).

PALS: Pulseless Electrical Activity (PEA)

Clinical Presentation

- Pediatric patient
- Unresponsive state
- No respirations or only agonal respirations
- Organized electrical rhythm on ECG monitor but no pulse
  1. Establish unresponsiveness with no respirations or only agonal respirations, no pulse. Call for help.
  2. **Begin CPR. Provide oxygen as soon as available.**
  3. Attach AED or monitor-defibrillator as soon as available without interrupting CPR. Use pediatric pads or paddles if available and indicated.
  4. When device is attached, stop CPR.
     - If using an AED and no shock is advised, immediately resume CPR beginning with compressions. Attach monitor-defibrillator as soon as available to assess rhythm.
     - If using a manual monitor-defibrillator, assess the rhythm. If rhythm is an organized rhythm, immediately resume CPR beginning with compressions.
  5. During CPR, establish IV or IO access.
     - Prepare vasopressor dose (epinephrine).
  6. Stop CPR. Assess rhythm.
  7. If PEA persists, administer epinephrine 0.01 mg/kg IV/IO (0.1 mL/kg of 1:10,000); follow with 20 mL IV flush.
     - Repeat every 3–5 min as needed.
     - If no IV/IO access is available and the patient has an ET in place, inject 0.1 mg/kg (0.1 mL/kg of 1:1,000) epinephrine directly into ET tube, followed by a 5-mL saline flush. Follow ET drug administration with ventilations to disperse drug into small airways for absorption into pulmonary vasculature.
  8. Insert an advanced airway (ET tube) if basic airway management is inadequate.
     - Confirm tube placement without interrupting CPR.
     - After correct placement is confirmed, deliver uninterrupted compressions at a rate of 100–120/min for 2 min and deliver 10 breaths/min at a rate of 1 breath every 6 sec.

164

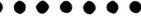

9. During CPR, consider and treat potentially reversible causes:

- Hypokalemia/hyperkalemia
- Hypovolemia
- Hypoxia or ventilation problems
- Hypoglycemia
- Hypothermia
- Hydrogen ion (acidosis)
- Tension pneumothorax
- Tamponade, cardiac
- Toxins
- Thrombosis (pulmonary or coronary)

10. Continue CPR; check the rhythm every 2 min.
11. If PEA persists, resume CPR and repeat steps 7, 9, and 10.
12. If rhythm becomes shockable with no pulse, follow VF/VT protocol.
13. If rhythm changes to asystole, follow asystole protocol.
14. If rhythm converts to a stable ECG rhythm with return of spontaneous circulation, monitor and reevaluate the patient. Arrange for transport to a critical care unit. The patient will need a comprehensive plan of care.

♥ **Clinical Tip:** PEA may be caused by potentially reversible conditions (Hs and Ts) and may be treated successfully if those conditions are identified and corrected early.

♥ **Clinical Tip:** When IV/IO access is not available, drugs may be delivered via an ET tube in the intubated patient. Stop CPR, administer the drug, flush with at least 5 mL normal saline, and deliver 5 consecutive positive-pressure ventilations to ensure proper drug delivery to the distal airways for absorption.

PALS: Asystole

Clinical Presentation

- Pediatric patient
- Unresponsive state
- No respirations or only agonal respirations
- No pulse
- Flat line or agonal rhythm, no electrical activity on ECG monitor
    1. Establish unresponsiveness with no respirations or only agonal respirations, no pulse. Call for help.
    2. Begin CPR. Provide oxygen as soon as available.

3. Attach AED or monitor-defibrillator as soon as available without interrupting CPR. Use pediatric pads or paddles if available and indicated.
4. When device is attached, stop CPR.
   - If using an AED and no shock is advised, immediately resume CPR beginning with compressions. Attach monitor-defibrillator as soon as available to assess rhythm.
   - If using a manual monitor-defibrillator, assess the rhythm. If there is no electrical activity (flat line or agonal rhythm), immediately resume CPR beginning with compressions.
5. During CPR, establish IV or IO access.
   - Prepare vasopressor dose (epinephrine).
6. Stop CPR. Assess rhythm.
7. If asystole persists, administer epinephrine 0.01 mg/kg IV/IO (0.1 mL/kg of 1:10,000); follow with 20-mL IV flush.
   - Repeat every 3–5 min as needed.
   - If no IV/IO access is available and the patient has an ET tube in place, inject 0.1 mg/kg (0.1 mL/kg of 1:1,000) epinephrine directly into ET tube, followed by a 5-mL saline flush. Follow ET drug administration with ventilations to disperse drug into small airways for absorption into pulmonary vasculature.
8. Insert an advanced airway (ET tube) if basic airway management is inadequate.
   - Confirm tube placement without interrupting CPR.
   - After correct placement is confirmed, deliver uninterrupted compressions at a rate of 100–120/min for 2 min and deliver 10 breaths/min at a rate of 1 breath every 6 sec.
9. During CPR consider and treat potentially reversible causes:
   - Hypokalemia/hyperkalemia
   - Hypovolemia
   - Hypoxia or ventilation problems
   - Hypoglycemia
   - Hypothermia
   - Hydrogen ion (acidosis)
   - Trauma (hypovolemia, increased ICP)
   - Tension pneumothorax
   - Tamponade, cardiac
   - Toxins
   - Thrombosis (pulmonary or coronary)

10. Continue CPR; check rhythm every 2 min.
11. If asystole persists, resume CPR and repeat steps 7, 9 and 10.
    - Consider whether proper resuscitation protocols were followed and reversible causes were identified.
    - If procedures were performed correctly, follow local criteria for terminating resuscitation efforts.
12. If rhythm is shockable with no pulse, follow VF/VT protocol.
13. If rhythm changes to an organized rhythm with no pulse, follow PEA protocol.
14. If rhythm converts to a stable ECG rhythm with return of spontaneous circulation, monitor and reevaluate the patient. Arrange for transport to a critical care unit. The patient will need a comprehensive plan of care.

♥ **Clinical Tip:** Emphasis must be on high-quality CPR, ensuring adequate rate and depth of chest compressions with complete chest recoil after each compression, minimizing interruptions in chest compressions (no more than 10 seconds when necessary), and avoiding excessive ventilation. Rotate chest compressor every 2 min to minimize fatigue.

♥ **Clinical Tip:** To calculate medication doses, use the pediatric patient's weight if known. If the weight is not known, use a pediatric body-length tape with precalculated doses, which are based on the 50th percentile of weight for length (ideal body weight) for a reasonable estimate of medication doses.

♥ **Clinical Tip:** Family presence during resuscitation may be beneficial to the family, providing an opportunity to say goodbye and facilitating the grieving process when resuscitation attempts are unsuccessful. Families should be offered this opportunity whenever possible.

PALS: Bradycardia

Clinical Presentation

- Pediatric patient
- Heart rate less than 60 bpm
- Respiratory distress or failure
- Signs of shock with hypotension, diaphoresis, altered mental status
    1. Establish responsiveness.
    2. Perform primary ABCDE survey.
    3. Measure vital signs, including oxygen saturation.
    4. Administer oxygen, establish IV/IO access, and attach monitor-defibrillator to identify rhythm.
    5. Obtain 12-lead ECG if possible for more accurate rhythm identification.
    6. Assess for signs and symptoms.
        - If the patient is stable and asymptomatic with a heart rate <60 bpm, support oxygenation and ventilation, monitor and observe for any changes, and seek expert consultation.
        - If the patient is symptomatic with a heart rate <60 bpm and signs of poor perfusion despite oxygenation and ventilation, perform CPR.
    7. If symptomatic bradycardia persists, administer epinephrine 0.01 mg/kg IV/IO (0.1 mL/kg of 1:10,000); follow with 20 mL IV flush.
        - Repeat every 3–5 min as needed.
        - If no IV/IO access is available and the patient has an ET tube in place, inject 0.1 mg/kg (0.1 mL/kg of 1:1,000) epinephrine directly into ET tube, followed by a 5-mL saline flush. Follow ET drug administration with ventilations to disperse drug into small airways for absorption into pulmonary vasculature.
    8. For increased vagal tone or primary AV block, administer a first dose of atropine 0.02 mg/kg IV/IO.
        - May repeat every 3–5 min. Minimum single dose 0.1 mg, maximum single dose 0.5 mg, maximum total dose 1 mg.
    9. If the patient fails to respond to atropine, consider transthoracic or transvenous pacing.
    10. Identify and treat the cause of bradycardia.

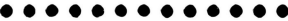

PALS: Tachycardia With Pulse, Narrow-Complex QRS (≤0.09 sec) With Adequate Perfusion

Clinical Presentation

- Pediatric patient
- Rapid heart rate
- No serious symptoms with signs of adequate perfusion
  1. Establish responsiveness.
  2. Perform primary ABCDE survey.
  3. Measure vital signs, including oxygen saturation.
  4. Administer oxygen, establish IV/IO access, and attach monitor-defibrillator to identify rhythm.
  5. Obtain a 12-lead ECG if possible for more accurate rhythm identification.
  6. Assess for signs and symptoms.
     - If the patient is stable and asymptomatic, with a heart rate less than 180 bpm for a child and less than 220 bpm for an infant, the rhythm is probably sinus tachycardia, not SVT. Search for and treat the underlying cause.
     - If the heart rate is ≥180 bpm for a child and ≥220 bpm for an infant, the rhythm is probably SVT; consider vagal maneuvers.
  7. If vagal maneuvers are ineffective and IV/IO access is available, give adenosine 0.1 mg/kg IV/IO rapid push.
     - Maximum first dose 6 mg.
     - May double the first dose and give 0.2 mg/kg IV/IO rapid push.
     - Maximum second dose 12 mg.
  8. Seek expert consultation. Search for and treat reversible causes.
  9. If rhythm has not converted to sinus, consider administration of amiodarone 5 mg/kg IV over 20–60 min or procainamide 15 mg/kg IV over 30–60 min.
     - Do not administer amiodarone and procainamide together.
  10. If medications are ineffective, or if patient becomes unstable, attempt synchronized cardioversion at 0.5–1.0 J/kg.
      - If unstable tachycardia persists, increase to 2 J/kg. Premedicate with a sedative plus an analgesic whenever possible but do not delay cardioversion.

PALS: Tachycardia With Pulse, Wide-Complex QRS (>0.09 sec) With Adequate Perfusion

Clinical Presentation

- Pediatric patient
- Rapid heart rate
- No serious symptoms with signs of adequate perfusion
  1. Establish responsiveness.
  2. Perform primary ABCDE survey.
  3. Measure vital signs, including oxygen saturation.
  4. Administer oxygen, establish IV/IO access, and attach monitor-defibrillator to identify rhythm.
  5. Obtain a 12-lead ECG if possible for more accurate rhythm identification.
  6. If rhythm is likely a supraventricular tachycardia with aberrancy (wide QRS), seek expert consultation.
     - Give adenosine 0.1 mg/kg IV/IO rapid push.
     - Maximum first dose 6 mg.
     - May double the first dose and give 0.2 mg/kg IV/IO rapid push.
     - Maximum second dose 12 mg.
     - Search for and treat reversible causes.
  7. If rhythm is likely ventricular tachycardia, seek expert consultation.
     - Prepare to administer amiodarone 5 mg/kg IV over 20-60 min or procainamide 15 mg/kg IV over 30–60 min. Do not administer amiodarone and procainamide together.
     - Search for and treat reversible causes.
  8. If medications are ineffective, or if patient becomes unstable, attempt synchronized cardioversion at 0.5–1.0 J/kg.
     - If unstable tachycardia persists, increase to 2 J/kg.
     - Premedicate with a sedative plus an analgesic whenever possible but do not delay cardioversion.

PALS: Tachycardia With Pulse, Narrow-Complex QRS (≤0.09 sec) With Poor Perfusion

Clinical Presentation

- Pediatric patient
- Altered LOC
- Shortness of breath, diaphoresis, fatigue, syncope, poor perfusion
  1. Establish responsiveness.
  2. Perform primary ABCDE survey.
  3. Measure vital signs, including oxygen saturation.
  4. Administer oxygen, establish IV/IO access, and attach monitor-defibrillator to identify rhythm.
  5. Obtain a 12-lead ECG if possible for more accurate rhythm identification.
  6. Assess for signs and symptoms.
     - If the patient is stable and asymptomatic, with a heart rate <180 bpm for a child and <220 bpm for an infant, normal P waves present and varying R-R intervals, the rhythm is probably sinus tachycardia, not SVT. Search for and treat the underlying cause.
     - If the heart rate is ≥180 bpm for a child and ≥220 bpm for an infant with absent P waves, regular rhythm and signs of poor perfusion, the rhythm is probably SVT; consider vagal maneuvers.
  7. If vagal maneuvers are ineffective and IV/IO access is available, give adenosine 0.1 mg/kg IV/IO rapid push.
     - Maximum first dose 6 mg.
     - May double first dose and give 0.2 mg/kg IV/IO rapid push.
     - Maximum second dose 12 mg.
     - Immediately follow each dose with 5- to 10-mL normal saline flush.
  8. If IV/IO access is not available or adenosine was ineffective, attempt synchronized cardioversion at 0.5–1.0 J/kg.
     - If unstable tachycardia persists, increase to 2 J/kg.
     - Premedicate with a sedative plus an analgesic whenever possible but do not delay cardioversion.

9. If cardioversion is unsuccessful, seek expert consultation.
10. Prepare to administer either amiodarone 5 mg/kg IV/IO over 20–60 min or procainamide 15 mg/kg IV/IO over 30–60 min.
   ■ Do not routinely administer amiodarone and procainamide together.

♥ **Clinical Tip:** If there are visible P waves with a constant PR interval and somewhat variable R-R intervals in an infant with a heart rate <220/min or a child with a heart rate <180/min, the rhythm is probably sinus tachycardia. The heart rate increases gradually rather than abruptly. Correlate with the pediatric patient's clinical history and always search for and treat the cause.

♥ **Clinical Tip:** If there are no visible P waves and therefore no measurable PR interval, with a regular R-R interval in an infant with a heart rate ≥220/min or a child with a heart rate ≥180/min, the rhythm is probably SVT. The rate typically changes abruptly. Treat according to the above algorithm.

PALS: Tachycardia With Pulse, Wide-Complex QRS (>0.09 sec) With Poor Perfusion

Clinical Presentation
■ Pediatric patient
■ Altered LOC
■ Shortness of breath, diaphoresis, fatigue, syncope, poor perfusion
   1. Establish responsiveness.
   2. Perform primary ABCDE survey.
   3. Measure vital signs, including oxygen saturation.
   4. Administer oxygen, establish IV/IO access, and attach monitor-defibrillator to identify rhythm.
   5. Obtain a 12-lead ECG if possible for more accurate rhythm identification.
   6. If the patient is experiencing cardiopulmonary compromise with a rapid heart rate and wide QRS complex, the rhythm is presumed to be ventricular tachycardia.
      ■ Prompt synchronized cardioversion is indicated.
      ■ Attempt synchronized cardioversion at 0.5–1 J/kg; if unstable tachycardia persists, increase to 2 J/kg.

172

- Premedicate with a sedative plus an analgesic whenever possible but do not delay cardioversion.

7. If the patient does not exhibit signs of cardiopulmonary compromise, consider adenosine if the wide-complex tachycardia is regular and monomorphic.
   - Give adenosine 0.1 mg/kg IV/IO rapid push (maximum first dose 6 mg).
   - May double the first dose and give 0.2 mg/kg IV/IO rapid push.
   - Maximum second dose 12 mg.

8. If cardioversion or adenosine is unsuccessful, seek expert consultation.

9. Prepare to administer either amiodarone 5 mg/kg IV/IO over 20–60 min or procainamide 15 mg/kg IV/IO over 30–60 min.
   - Do not routinely administer amiodarone and procainamide together.

♥ **Clinical Tip:** Wide-complex tachycardia is a relatively uncommon rhythm in children; however, it can be seen in children with heart disease, drug ingestion (tricyclic antidepressants), and hyperkalemia.

PALS: Immediate Post–Cardiac Arrest Care

1. Upon return of spontaneous circulation, assess responsiveness, perform primary ABCDE survey and secondary assessment. Measure vital signs, including oxygen saturation.

2. Airway, breathing:
   - Provide oxygen to maintain oxygen saturation 94%–99% for optimal oxygenation.
   - Wean oxygen within the range of 94%–99% if oxygen is 100% to prevent hyperoxemia and associated oxidative injury.
   - Unless awake and alert, the patient may require an advanced airway and monitoring with waveform capnography.
   - Hyperventilation must be avoided. Target end-tidal CO_2 should be 35–40 mm Hg.

3. Circulation:
   - Assess for presence of shock.
   - Treat persistent shock with 20 mL/kg IV/IO boluses of normal saline or lactated Ringer's. Consider smaller boluses (10 mL/kg) if poor cardiac function is suspected.
   - If hypotensive shock persists, consider vasopressor infusion with epinephrine, dopamine, or norepinephrine.
   - If normotensive shock, consider dobutamine, dopamine, epinephrine, or milrinone.

4. Consider and treat potentially reversible causes of cardiac arrest:
   - Hypokalemia/hyperkalemia
   - Hypovolemia
   - Hypoxia or ventilation problems
   - Hypoglycemia
   - Hypothermia
   - Hydrogen ion (acidosis)
   - Trauma (hypovolemia, increased ICP)
   - Tension pneumothorax
   - Tamponade, cardiac
   - Toxins
   - Thrombosis (pulmonary or coronary)

5. Obtain a chest radiograph to confirm ET tube placement, assess pulmonary status, and evaluate heart size.

6. Obtain a 12-lead ECG as soon as possible.

7. For patients who are comatose in the first several days after cardiac arrest, temperature should be monitored continuously and fever should be treated aggressively.

8. If the patient remains comatose, maintain Targeted Temperature Management (TTM) for either 5 days of normalthermia (36°C–37.5°C) or 2 days of continuous hypothermia (32°C–34°C) followed by 3 days of normothermia.

9. Monitor the patient for pain, agitation, and seizures; initiate appropriate treatment if present.

10. Monitor the patient for hypoglycemia and initiate appropriate treatment if present.

11. Advanced critical care with development of a comprehensive plan of care should be provided to all survivors of cardiac arrest to optimize neurological, cardiopulmonary, and metabolic function.

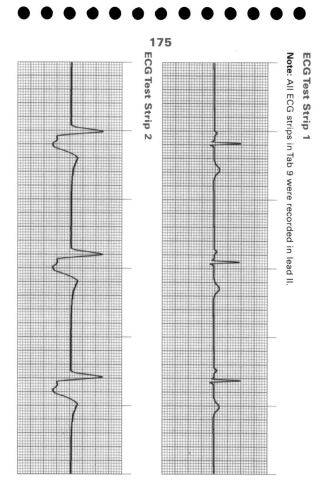

ECG Test Strip 1

Note: All ECG strips in Tab 9 were recorded in lead II.

ECG Test Strip 2

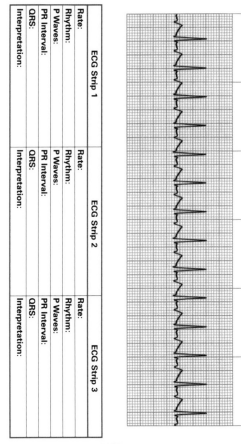

ECG Strip 1	ECG Strip 2	ECG Strip 3
Rate:	Rate:	Rate:
Rhythm:	Rhythm:	Rhythm:
P Waves:	P Waves:	P Waves:
PR Interval:	PR Interval:	PR Interval:
QRS:	QRS:	QRS:
Interpretation:	Interpretation:	Interpretation:

Case Study One: A 66-year-old woman with a history of heart disease is found unresponsive. This is an unwitnessed cardiac arrest with the initial rhythm shown in ECG strip 4. CPR is initiated while the defibrillator is charged. Strip 5 shows the rhythm following defibrillation. Because the first defibrillation was unsuccessful, the machine is charged a second time. The next rhythm is shown in strip 6.

ECG Strip 4 Interpretation:

ECG Strip 5 Interpretation:

ECG Strip 6 Interpretation:

ECG Test Strip 4

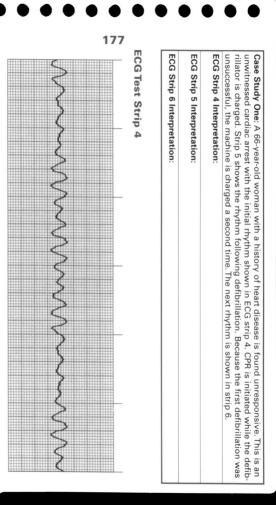

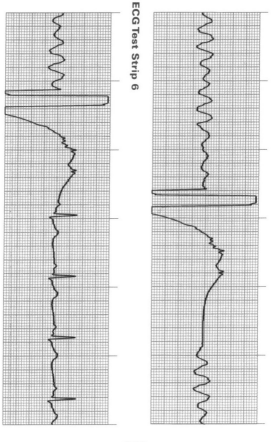

ECG Test Strip 5

ECG Test Strip 6

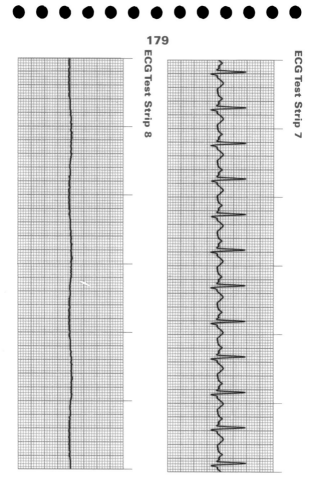

ECG Test Strip 8

ECG Test Strip 7

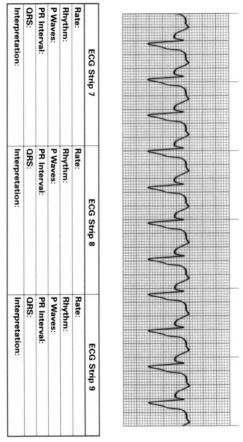

ECG Test Strip 9

ECG Strip 7		ECG Strip 8		ECG Strip 9
Rate:		Rate:		Rate:
Rhythm:		Rhythm:		Rhythm:
P Waves:		P Waves:		P Waves:
PR Interval:		PR Interval:		PR Interval:
QRS:		QRS:		QRS:
Interpretation:		Interpretation:		Interpretation:

Case Study Two: A 72-year-old man is complaining of dizziness and anxiety. Strip 10 shows his initial rhythm. An IV is started, and the patient is given oxygen, but his vital signs become unstable (strip 11). An IVP of adenosine is given, and his condition stabilizes with the final rhythm, shown in strip 12.

ECG Strip 10 Interpretation:

ECG Strip 11 Interpretation:

ECG Strip 12 Interpretation:

ECG Test Strip 10

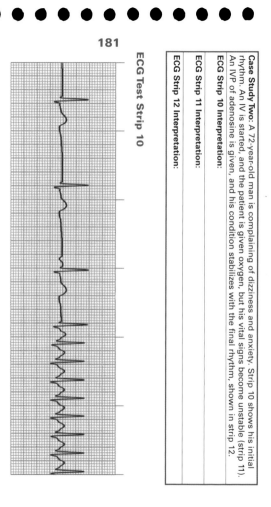

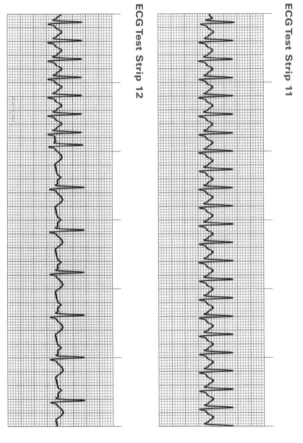

ECG Test Strip 11

ECG Test Strip 12

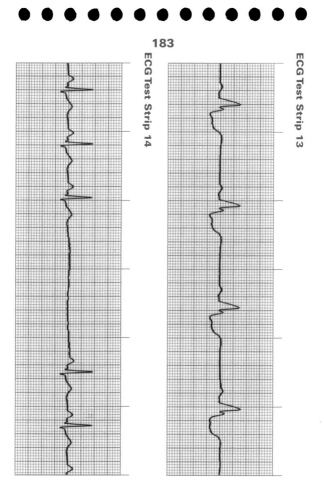

ECG Test Strip 14

ECG Test Strip 13

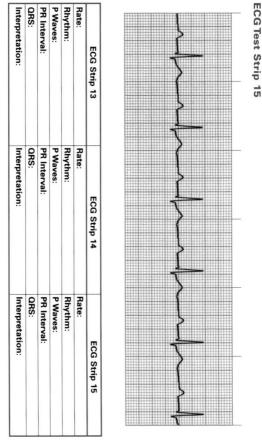

	ECG Strip 13		ECG Strip 14		ECG Strip 15
Rate:		Rate:		Rate:	
Rhythm:		Rhythm:		Rhythm:	
P Waves:		P Waves:		P Waves:	
PR Interval:		PR Interval:		PR Interval:	
QRS:		QRS:		QRS:	
Interpretation:		Interpretation:		Interpretation:	

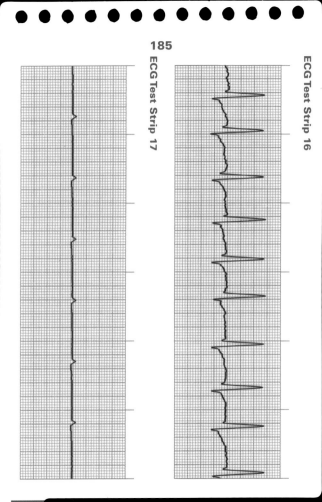

ECG Test Strip 16

ECG Test Strip 17

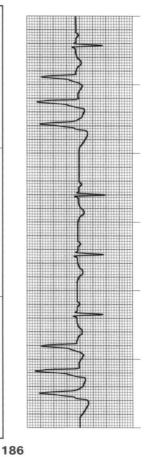

ECG Strip 16	ECG Strip 17	ECG Strip 18
Rate:	Rate:	Rate:
Rhythm:	Rhythm:	Rhythm:
P Waves:	P Waves:	P Waves:
PR Interval:	PR Interval:	PR Interval:
QRS:	QRS:	QRS:
Interpretation:	Interpretation:	Interpretation:

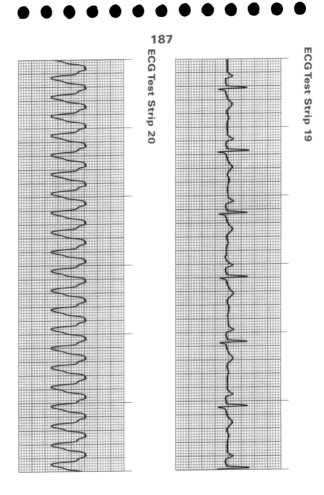

ECG Test Strip 20

ECG Test Strip 19

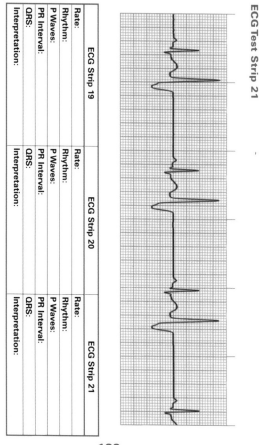

ECG Strip 19		ECG Strip 20		ECG Strip 21
Rate:		**Rate:**		**Rate:**
Rhythm:		**Rhythm:**		**Rhythm:**
P Waves:		**P Waves:**		**P Waves:**
PR Interval:		**PR Interval:**		**PR Interval:**
QRS:		**QRS:**		**QRS:**
Interpretation:		**Interpretation:**		**Interpretation:**

ECG Test Strip 22

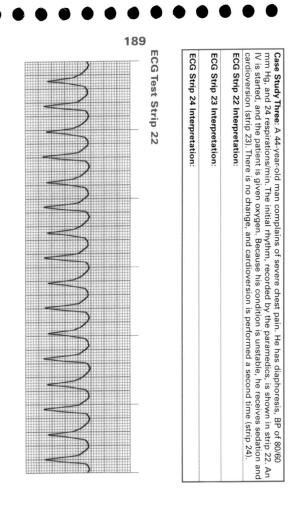

Case Study Three: A 44-year-old man complains of severe chest pain. He has diaphoresis, BP of 80/60 mm Hg, and 24 respirations/min. The initial rhythm, recorded by the paramedics, is shown in strip 22. An IV is started, and the patient is given oxygen. Because his condition is unstable, he receives sedation and cardioversion (strip 23). There is no change, and cardioversion is performed a second time (strip 24).

ECG Strip 22 Interpretation:

ECG Strip 23 Interpretation:

ECG Strip 24 Interpretation:

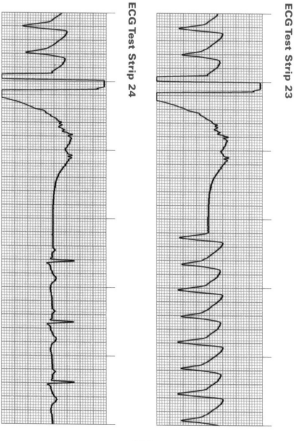

ECG Test Strip 24

ECG Test Strip 23

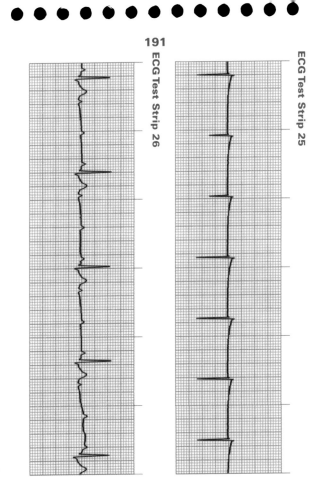

ECG Test Strip 26

ECG Test Strip 25

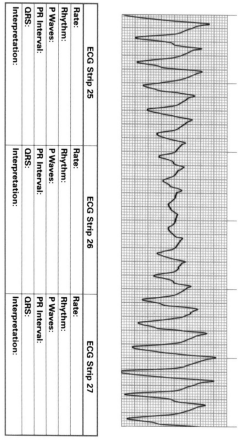

ECG Test Strip 27

ECG Strip 25		ECG Strip 26		ECG Strip 27	
Rate:		Rate:		Rate:	
Rhythm:		Rhythm:		Rhythm:	
P Waves:		P Waves:		P Waves:	
PR Interval:		PR Interval:		PR Interval:	
QRS:		QRS:		QRS:	
Interpretation:		Interpretation:		Interpretation:	

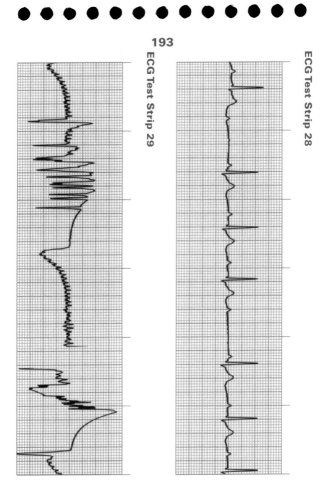

ECG Test Strip 29

ECG Test Strip 28

ECG Test Strip 30

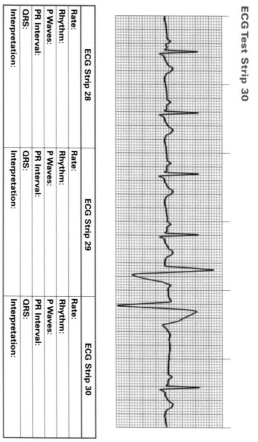

ECG Strip 28		ECG Strip 29		ECG Strip 30
Rate:		**Rate:**		**Rate:**
Rhythm:		**Rhythm:**		**Rhythm:**
P Waves:		**P Waves:**		**P Waves:**
PR Interval:		**PR Interval:**		**PR Interval:**
QRS:		**QRS:**		**QRS:**
Interpretation:		**Interpretation:**		**Interpretation:**

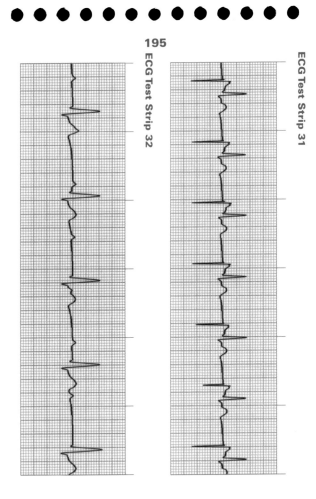

ECG Test Strip 32

ECG Test Strip 31

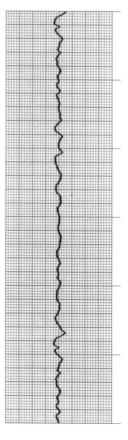

ECG Strip 31	ECG Strip 32	ECG Strip 33
Rate:	Rate:	Rate:
Rhythm:	Rhythm:	Rhythm:
P Waves:	P Waves:	P Waves:
PR Interval:	PR Interval:	PR Interval:
QRS:	QRS:	QRS:
Interpretation:	Interpretation:	Interpretation:

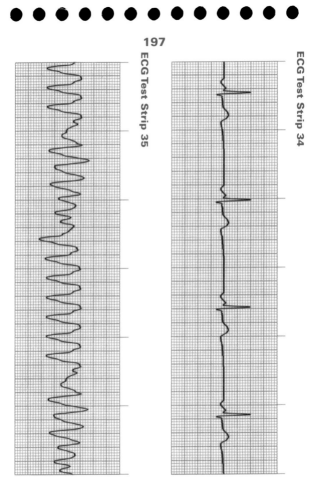

ECG Test Strip 35

ECG Test Strip 34

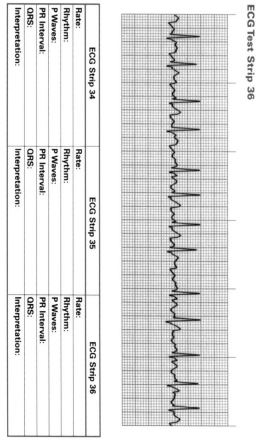

ECG Test Strip 36

ECG Strip 34		ECG Strip 35		ECG Strip 36
Rate:		**Rate:**		**Rate:**
Rhythm:		**Rhythm:**		**Rhythm:**
P Waves:		**P Waves:**		**P Waves:**
PR Interval:		**PR Interval:**		**PR Interval:**
QRS:		**QRS:**		**QRS:**
Interpretation:		**Interpretation:**		**Interpretation:**

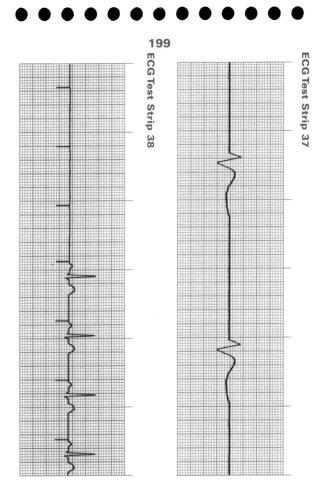

ECG Test Strip 38

ECG Test Strip 37

ECG Test Strip 39

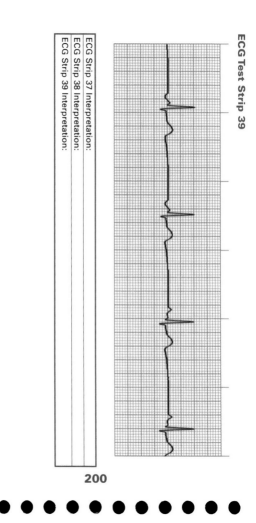

ECG Strip 37 Interpretation:

ECG Strip 38 Interpretation:

ECG Strip 39 Interpretation:

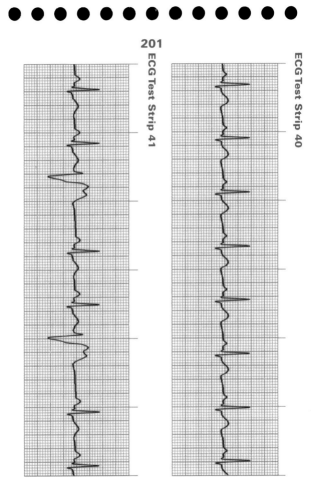

ECG Test Strip 41

ECG Test Strip 40

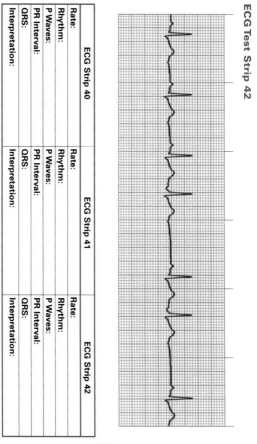

ECG Test Strip 42

ECG Strip 40	ECG Strip 41	ECG Strip 42
Rate:	Rate:	Rate:
Rhythm:	Rhythm:	Rhythm:
P Waves:	P Waves:	P Waves:
PR Interval:	PR Interval:	PR Interval:
QRS:	QRS:	QRS:
Interpretation:	Interpretation:	Interpretation:

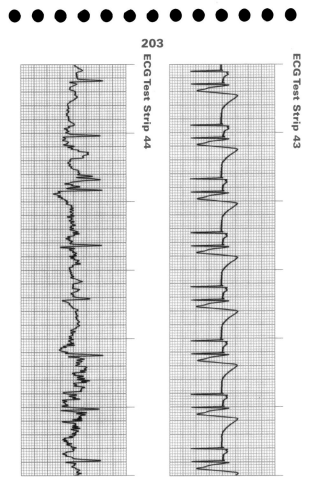

203

ECG Test Strip 44

ECG Test Strip 43

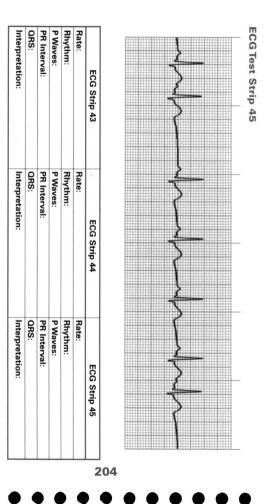

ECG Test Strip 45

ECG Strip 43		ECG Strip 44		ECG Strip 45
Rate:		Rate:		Rate:
Rhythm:		Rhythm:		Rhythm:
P Waves:		P Waves:		P Waves:
PR Interval:		PR Interval:		PR Interval:
QRS:		QRS:		QRS:
Interpretation:		Interpretation:		Interpretation:

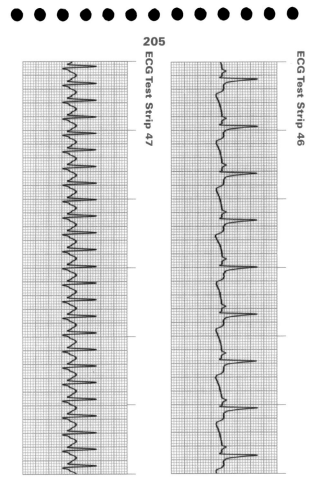

ECG Test Strip 47

ECG Test Strip 46

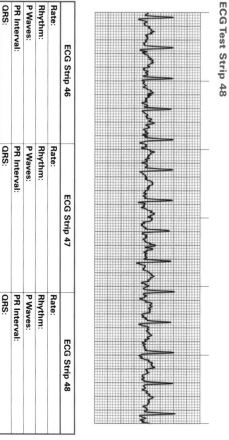

ECG Strip 46	ECG Strip 47	ECG Strip 48
Rate:	Rate:	Rate:
Rhythm:	Rhythm:	Rhythm:
P Waves:	P Waves:	P Waves:
PR Interval:	PR Interval:	PR Interval:
QRS:	QRS:	QRS:
Interpretation:	Interpretation:	Interpretation:

206

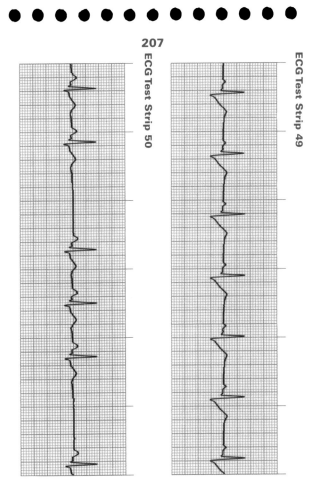

ECG Test Strip 50

ECG Test Strip 49

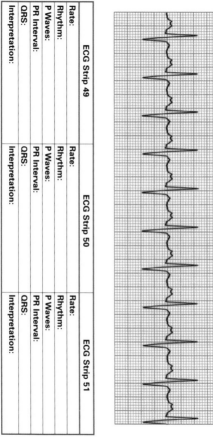

ECG Strip 49	ECG Strip 50	ECG Strip 51
Rate:	Rate:	Rate:
Rhythm:	Rhythm:	Rhythm:
P Waves:	P Waves:	P Waves:
PR Interval:	PR Interval:	PR Interval:
QRS:	QRS:	QRS:
Interpretation:	Interpretation:	Interpretation:

208

Answers to ECG Test Strips

	ECG Strip 1	ECG Strip 2	ECG Strip 3
Rate: 35 bpm		**Rate:** 34 bpm	**Rate:** Ventricular 150 bpm, atrial 280 bpm
Rhythm: Regular		**Rhythm:** Regular	**Rhythm:** Regular
P Waves: Normal		**P Waves:** None	**P Waves:** Flutter waves
PR Interval: 0.16 sec		**PR Interval:** None	**PR Interval:** Variable
QRS: 0.10 sec		**QRS:** 0.20 sec	**QRS:** 0.08 sec
Interpretation: Sinus bradycardia		**Interpretation:** Idioventricular rhythm	**Interpretation:** Atrial flutter with 2:1 conduction

ECG Strip 4 Interpretation: Ventricular fibrillation

ECG Strip 5 Interpretation: VF with defibrillation converting back to same rhythm

ECG Strip 6 Interpretation: VF with defibrillation converting to sinus rhythm at 68 bpm

	ECG Strip 7	ECG Strip 8	ECG Strip 9
Rate: 115 bpm		**Rate:** None	**Rate:** 115 bpm
Rhythm: Regular		**Rhythm:** None	**Rhythm:** Regular
P Waves: Normal		**P Waves:** None	**P Waves:** None
PR Interval: 0.12 sec		**PR Interval:** None	**PR Interval:** None
QRS: 0.10 sec		**QRS:** None	**QRS:** Wide (>0.12 sec), bizarre
Interpretation: Sinus tachycardia		**Interpretation:** Asystole	**Interpretation:** Ventricular tachycardia—monomorphic

ECG Strip 10 Interpretation: Paroxysmal supraventricular tachycardia—initial junctional rhythm at 48 bpm, converting to supraventricular tachycardia at 250 bpm

ECG Strip 11 Interpretation: SVT at 250 bpm

ECG Strip 12 Interpretation: SVT at 250 bpm converting to a sinus rhythm at 100 bpm

ECG Strip 13	ECG Strip 14	ECG Strip 15
Rate: 41 bpm	**Rate:** Basic rate 79 bpm	**Rate:** 58 bpm
Rhythm: Regular	**Rhythm:** Irregular	**Rhythm:** Regular
P Waves: Normal	**P Waves:** Normal	**P Waves:** Normal
PR Interval: 0.20 sec	**PR Interval:** 0.16 sec	**PR Interval:** 0.32 sec
QRS: 0.24 sec	**QRS:** 0.08 sec	**QRS:** 0.08 sec
Interpretation: Sinus bradycardia with a bundle branch block	**Interpretation:** Sinus rhythm with sinus pause/arrest	**Interpretation:** Sinus bradycardia with first-degree AV block

ECG Strip 16	ECG Strip 17	ECG Strip 18
Rate: Atrial >350 bpm, ventricular 88–115 bpm	**Rate:** Atrial 60 bpm	**Rate:** Basic rate 68 bpm
Rhythm: Irregular	**Rhythm:** Atrial regular	**Rhythm:** Irregular
P Waves: None	**P Waves:** Normal	**P Waves:** Normal
PR Interval: None	**PR Interval:** None	**PR Interval:** 0.16 sec
QRS: 0.12 sec	**QRS:** None	**QRS:** 0.08 sec
Interpretation: Atrial fibrillation	**Interpretation:** P Wave asystole	**Interpretation:** Sinus rhythm with premature ventricular contractions—triplets

ECG Strip 19	ECG Strip 20	ECG Strip 21
Rate: 65 bpm	**Rate:** 214 bpm	**Rate:** Basic rate 35 bpm
Rhythm: Regular	**Rhythm:** Regular	**Rhythm:** Regular
P Waves: Normal	**P Waves:** None	**P Waves:** Normal
PR Interval: 0.20 sec	**PR Interval:** None	**PR Interval:** 0.16 sec
QRS: 0.08 sec	**QRS:** Wide (>0.12 sec), bizarre	**QRS:** 0.08 sec
Interpretation: Normal sinus rhythm with U wave	**Interpretation:** VT— monomorphic	**Interpretation:** Sinus bradycardia with ventricular bigeminy

---

ECG Strip 22 Interpretation: VT—monomorphic

ECG Strip 23 Interpretation: VT—monomorphic with cardioversion converting to same rhythm

ECG Strip 24 Interpretation: VT—monomorphic with cardioversion converting to a sinus rhythm at 65 bpm

---

ECG Strip 25	ECG Strip 26	ECG Strip 27
Rate: Pacing spikes 68 bpm	**Rate:** Atrial 125 bpm, ventricular 44 bpm	**Rate:** 200–250 bpm
Rhythm: Regular pacing spikes	**Rhythm:** Regular	**Rhythm:** Irregular
P Waves: None	**P Waves:** Normal	**P Waves:** None
PR Interval: None	**PR Interval:** 0.16 sec	**PR Interval:** None
QRS: None	**QRS:** 0.10 sec	**QRS:** Wide (>0.12 sec), bizarre
Interpretation: Pacemaker— 100% failure to capture; underlying rhythm asystole	**Interpretation:** Second-degree AV block type II with 3:1 conduction	**Interpretation:** VT—torsade de pointes

ECG Strip 28		ECG Strip 29		ECG Strip 30
Rate: 50–75 bpm		**Rate**: None		**Rate**: Basic rate 68 bpm
Rhythm: Irregular		**Rhythm**: None		**Rhythm**: Irregular
P Waves: Normal		**P Waves**: None		**P Waves**: Normal
PR Interval: 0.12–0.28 sec		**PR Interval**: None		**PR Interval**: 0.16 sec
QRS: 0.08 sec		**QRS**: None		**QRS**: 0.10 sec
Interpretation: Second-degree AV block type I		**Interpretation**: Loose electrodes		**Interpretation**: Sinus rhythm with multiform PVCs—couplets

ECG Strip 31		ECG Strip 32		ECG Strip 33
Rate: 68 bpm		**Rate**: Atrial 75 bpm, ventricular 48 bpm		**Rate**: Indeterminate
Rhythm: Regular		**Rhythm**: Regular		**Rhythm**: Irregular
P Waves: Upright with pacing spikes		**P Waves**: Normal, superimposed on QRS and T waves		**P Waves**: None
PR Interval: 0.16 sec		**PR Interval**: Varies		**PR Interval**: None
QRS: 0.10 sec		**QRS**: 0.16 sec		**QRS**: None
Interpretation: Atrial pacemaker with 100% capture		**Interpretation**: Third-degree AV block		**Interpretation**: VF

ECG Strip 34	ECG Strip 35	ECG Strip 36
Rate: 48 bpm	**Rate:** 250 bpm	**Rate:** Atrial ≥350 bpm, ventricular 94–167 bpm
Rhythm: Regular	**Rhythm:** Irregular	**Rhythm:** Irregular
P Waves: Inverted	**P Waves:** None	**P Waves:** None
PR Interval: 0.12 sec	**PR Interval:** None	**PR Interval:** None
QRS: 0.08 sec	**QRS:** Wide (>0.12 sec), bizarre	**QRS:** 0.10 sec
Interpretation: Junctional rhythm	**Interpretation:** VT—polymorphic	**Interpretation:** A-fib

ECG Strip 37 Interpretation: Agonal rhythm at 22 bpm

ECG Strip 38 Interpretation: Pacemaker failure to capture. When the pacemaker voltage is increased, there is capture at pacemaker spike 4.

ECG Strip 39 Interpretation: Junctional bradycardia at 38 bpm converting to sinus bradycardia at 38 bpm

ECG Strip 40	ECG Strip 41	ECG Strip 42
Rate: 75 bpm	**Rate:** Basic rate 79 bpm	**Rate:** Basic rate 68 bpm
Rhythm: Regular	**Rhythm:** Irregular	**Rhythm:** Irregular
P Waves: Normal	**P Waves:** Normal	**P Waves:** Normal; none associated with premature junctional contraction
PR Interval: 0.16 sec	**PR Interval:** 0.20 sec	**PR Interval:** 0.16 sec
QRS: 0.08 sec	**QRS:** 0.10 sec	**QRS:** 0.10 sec
Interpretation: Normal sinus rhythm	**Interpretation:** Sinus rhythm with ventricular trigeminy	**Interpretation:** Sinus rhythm with PJCs at beats 4 and 6

ECG Strip 43	ECG Strip 44	ECG Strip 45
Rate: 75 bpm	**Rate:** 75 bpm	**Rate:** 68 bpm
Rhythm: Regular	**Rhythm:** Regular	**Rhythm:** Irregular
P Waves: Upright with pacing spike	**P Waves:** Not visible	**P Waves:** Normal
PR Interval: 0.20 sec	**PR Interval:** Not measurable	**PR Interval:** 0.16 sec
QRS: 0.16 sec	**QRS:** Not measurable	**QRS:** 0.10 sec
Interpretation: Atrial-ventricular pacemaker	**Interpretation:** Sinus rhythm with muscle artifact	**Interpretation:** Sinus rhythm with two premature atrial contractions (beats 2 and 7)

ECG Strip 46	ECG Strip 47	ECG Strip 48
Rate: 88 bpm	**Rate:** 250 bpm	**Rate:** 136 bpm
Rhythm: Regular	**Rhythm:** Regular	**Rhythm:** Regular
P Waves: Normal	**P Waves:** Buried in T waves	**P Waves:** Not visible
PR Interval: 0.12 sec	**PR Interval:** Not measurable	**PR Interval:** Not measurable
QRS: 0.12 sec	**QRS:** 0.08 sec	**QRS:** 0.10 sec
Interpretation: Sinus rhythm with ST segment elevation	**Interpretation:** SVT	**Interpretation:** Sinus tachycardia with muscle artifact

ECG Strip 49	ECG Strip 50	ECG Strip 51
Rate: 71 bpm	**Rate:** Basic rate 79 bpm	**Rate:** 107 bpm
Rhythm: Regular	**Rhythm:** Irregular	**Rhythm:** Regular
P Waves: Normal	**P Waves:** Normal	**P Waves:** Notched (P prime)
PR Interval: 0.16 sec	**PR Interval:** 0.16 sec	**PR Interval:** 0.20 sec
QRS: 0.10 sec	**QRS:** 0.10 sec	**QRS:** 0.12 sec
Interpretation: Sinus rhythm with ST segment depression	**Interpretation:** Sinus rhythm with two SA blocks	**Interpretation:** Sinus tachycardia with P prime wave

Notes:

Troubleshooting ECG Problems

Without proper assessment and treatment, a patient with an abnormal ECG could have a potentially fatal outcome. An accurate and properly monitored ECG is extremely important, so remember the following troubleshooting tips:

- Place leads in the correct position. Incorrect placement can give false readings.
- Avoid placing leads over bony areas.
- In patients with large breasts, place the electrodes under the breast. The most accurate tracings are obtained through the smallest amount of fat tissue.
- Apply tincture of benzoin to the electrode sites if the patient is diaphoretic. The electrodes will adhere to the skin better.
- Shave hair at the electrode site if it interferes with contact between the electrode and the skin.
- Discard old electrodes and use new ones if the gel on the back of the electrode dries.

Cable Connections

- It is important to know whether you are using an American or a European cable for ECG monitoring. The colors of the wires differ, as shown below.

Monitoring Cable Connections		
U.S.	Connect to	Europe
White	Right arm	Red
Black	Left arm	Yellow
Red	Left leg	Green
Green	Right leg	Black
Brown	Chest	White

Patient Cable

- Monitoring cables contain varying numbers of wires.
- 3- and 4-wire cables: Allow a choice of limb and augmented leads.
- 5-wire cable: Allows a choice of limb and augmented leads plus a chest lead.
- 10-wire cable: Records a 12-lead ECG.

Patient ECG Record

Patient Name: _____

Sex: Female   **Male**

Heart Rate: _____ bpm

- Normal (60–100 bpm): Y   N
- Bradycardia (<60 bpm): Y   N
- Tachycardia (>100 bpm): Y   N

Rhythm

- Regular: Y   N
- Irregular: Y   N
- P waves: Y   N

P waves

- Normal (upright and uniform): Y   N
- Inverted: Y   N
- P wave associated with QRS complex: Y   N
- PR interval normal (0.12–0.20 sec): Y   N
- P waves and QRS complexes associated with one another: Y   N

QRS complex

- Normal (0.06–0.10 sec): Y   N
- Wide (>0.10 sec): Y   N

Are the QRS complexes grouped or not grouped?

Are there any dropped beats?

Is there a compensatory or noncompensatory pause?

QT interval: _____

Interpretation: _____

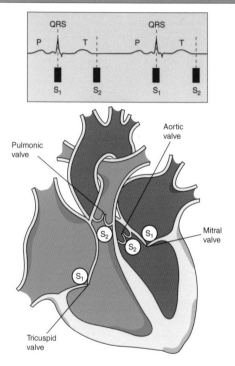

HEART RATE 2 Cycles from reference arrow (25 mm/s)

30 · 35 · 40 · 45 · 50 · 55 · 60 65 · 70 75 80 · 90 100 · 125 150 · 200 · 300 400

HEART RATE 1 Cycle from reference arrow (25 mm/s)

150 125 · 100 · 80 75 · 65 60 · 55 50 · 45 · 40 · 35 · 30 · 27 25 · 23 · 21 20 · 19 18 · 17 16

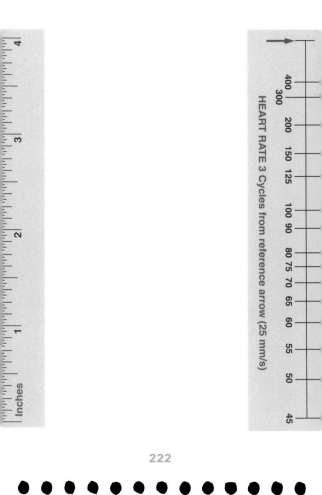

Inches 1 2 3 4

HEART RATE 3 Cycles from reference arrow (25 mm/s)

45 50 55 60 65 70 75 80 90 100 125 150 200 300 400

Abbreviations

ACE ......angiotensin-converting enzyme
ACLS .....advanced cardiac life support
ACS ......acute coronary syndrome
AED ......automatic external defibrillator
A-fib ......atrial fibrillation
A-flutter . . .atrial flutter
AV ....atrioventricular
BBB ......bundle branch block
BP ....blood pressure
bpm ......beats per minute
BUN ......blood urea nitrogen
CHF ......congestive heart failure
CO ....cardiac output
COPD .....chronic obstructive pulmonary disease
CPR ....cardiopulmonary resuscitation
CT ....computed tomography
ECG ......electrocardiogram
EMD ......electromechanical dissociation
ET ....endotracheal
FAB ......fragment antigen binding
gtt ....drops
HR ....heart rate
HTN ......hypertension
IHSS ......idiopathic hypertrophic subaortic stenosis
IM ....intramuscular
IO ....intraosseous
IV ....intravenous
LA ....left arm
LL ....left leg
LMA .....laryngeal mask airway
LOC ......level of consciousness
MAT ......multifocal atrial tachycardia
MCL ......modified chest lead
MI ....myocardial infarction
NSR ......normal sinus rhythm
PAC ......premature atrial contraction
PALS ......pediatric advanced life support
PAT ....paroxysmal atrial tachycardia

PEA . . . . . . .pulseless electrical activity
PJC . . . . . . .premature junctional contraction
PO . . . . .by mouth
PSVT . . . . .paroxysmal supraventricular tachycardia
PVC . . . . . . .premature ventricular contraction
QTc . . . . . . .QT interval corrected for heart rate
RA . . . . .right arm
RL . . . . .right leg
SA . . . . .sinoatrial
SV . . . . .stroke volume
SVT . . . . . . .supraventricular tachycardia
TKO . . . . . .to keep open
VF . . . . .ventricular fibrillation
VT . . . . .ventricular tachycardia
WAP . . . . . .wandering atrial pacemaker
WPW . . . . .Wolff-Parkinson-White (syndrome)

Selected References

1. American Heart Association: Basic Life Support for Healthcare Providers (Student Manual). American Heart Association, Dallas, TX, 2015.
2. American Heart Association: Guidelines for Cardiopulmonary Resuscitation and Emergency Cardiovascular Care. Supplement to Circulation 132 (18), November 3, 2015.
3. Deglin, JH, Vallerand, AH: Davis's Drug Guide for Nurses, ed 13. F. A. Davis, Philadelphia, 2013.
4. Jones, SA: Author's personal collection.
5. Jones, SA: ECG Notes, ed 1. F. A. Davis, Philadelphia, 2005.
6. Jones, SA: ECG Success. F. A. Davis, Philadelphia, 2008.
7. Myers, E: RNotes, ed 3. F. A. Davis, Philadelphia, 2010.
8. Hopkins, T: MedSurg Notes, ed 3. F. A. Davis, Philadelphia, 2011.
9. Scanlon, VC, Sanders, T: Essentials of Anatomy and Physiology, ed 6. F. A. Davis, Philadelphia, 2011.

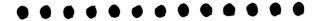

Illustration Credits

ECG strips on pages 28, 32–70, 73–78, 152–185 from Jones, SA: Author's personal collection.

Pages 10, 12, 13 from Jones, SA: ECG Success. F. A. Davis, Philadelphia, 2008.

Pages 14, 109, 123 from Myers, E: RNotes, ed 2. F. A. Davis, Philadelphia, 2006.

Pages 19, 81, 112, 127, 197 from Myers, E, Hopkins, T: MedSurg Notes. F. A. Davis, Philadelphia, 2004.

Pages 11, 22 adapted from Myers, E, Hopkins, T: MedSurg Notes. F. A. Davis, Philadelphia, 2004.

Pages 2, 3, 4, 5, 6, 7, 8 from Scanlon, VC, Sanders, T: Essentials of Anatomy and Physiology, ed 4. F. A. Davis, Philadelphia, 2003.

Index